TRAINING DISABLED
PEOPLE

SARA WICEBLOOM

A & C BLACK · LONDON

Thanks to Fitness Professionals Ltd (www.fitpro.com) for supporting the Fitness Professionals series

Note

It is always the responsibility of the individual to assess his or her own fitness capability before participating in any training activity. Whilst every effort has been made to ensure the content of this book is as technically accurate as possible, neither the author nor the publishers can accept responsibility for any injury or loss sustained as a result of the use of this material.

First published 2007 by A&C Black Publishers Ltd
38 Soho Square, London W1D 3HB
www.acblack.com

ISBN 978-0-713679-23-6

A CIP catalogue record for this book is available from the British Library.

Typeset in Berthold Baskerville Regular by Palimpsest Book Production Limited, Grangemouth, Stirlingshire

Cover image © Inclusive Fitness Initiative, reproduced with kind permission. For more information on the work of the IFI, please go to www.inclusivefitness.org.

Inside photographs © Grant Pritchard, except P103 © Alex Hazle.
Image on page 102 © RNID, reproduced with kind permission.

Printed and bound in Great Britain by Biddles Ltd, Kings Lynn, Norfolk

A&C Black uses paper produced with elemental chlorine-free pulp, harvested from managed sustainable forests.

CONTENTS

HOW TO USE THIS BOOK

It is generally recognised that the rewards to be gained from participation in fitness activities can be enormous. Not only are there the health benefits that we know regular physical activity can bring, but also benefits from tangible improvements to everyday life. Disabled people may indeed have more to gain from their participation, as some are at a greater risk of developing further (secondary) diseases, and some find difficulties in tackling the physical demands of everyday life.

Yet until very recently disabled people were not encouraged to attend fitness facilities. In fact they were often actively discouraged from it, mainly because of a lack of suitable equipment and facilities. Despite this focus on equipment and facilities, success stories about fitness experiences have more to do with the quality of service received from the instructors than with the leisure centre environment. As Chris Holmes, Paralympic gold medallist, has said, it's all about 'changing attitudes so that people, both disabled and non-disabled, have a really positive experience'.

I have heard time and time again how fear prevents some instructors from approaching disabled people – a fear of saying or doing the 'wrong' thing. This book seeks to dispel these fears. It provides information and advice in one user-friendly resource, to enable instructors to expand upon current good practice and to be inclusive, with a 'can do' approach to their work.

The book is split into three parts:

- **Part one** sets the scene by stating exactly who we are talking about when we use the term 'disabled people', and then presents information on the benefits of physical activity, the structures currently in place to support fitness provision for disabled people, and finally health and safety guidelines.
- **Part two** provides generalised information on how to work with disabled people, explaining the barriers that many face in their access to fitness activities and how fitness instructors can help to engage their disabled clients in meaningful physical activity.
- **Part three** provides guidelines for inclusive exercise programming with disabled people. This includes key information and exercise principles relating to specific medical conditions.

Parts two and three provide tips, photographs and real-life practical examples in the form of case studies, to help support the theory.

Using scientific research where it exists, the content encourages analysis and application according to each individual's physiology (body), psychology (mind/personality) and sociology (environment). The information and advice given should provide no more than a basis for further client consultation, as it is important to remember that each and every person is an individual.

The book covers the knowledge required for completing N/SVQ unit D442, which is designed for preparing advanced instructors to work with disabled clients (*see* table 0.1).

I hope that after reading this book, you and the disabled people with whom you work will enjoy and be rewarded by your shared fitness experience.

Table 0.1	N/SVQ Unit D442: Adapt a physical activity programme to the needs of disabled clients

What you must know and understand:
- The basic requirements of legislation relating to disability.
- The value of physical activity to clients with physical disability, learning difficulties and sensory impairment.
- The importance of working with disabled clients in a way that helps them achieve their full potential.
- The limits of your own competence and those of other professionals when working with disabled clients.
- Considerations when establishing and developing an effective working relationship with disabled clients and, where appropriate, their carers.
- The types of attitudes and misconceptions that you and others may have towards disabled clients and the importance of being accepting and non-judgemental.
- Common physical and psychological barriers to physical activity that disabled clients may face and how to respond to these barriers in a way that will motivate and involve clients.

- Basic features of the following types of impairments including:
  - arthritis
  - amputation
  - sensory (visual, auditory)
  - learning difficulties
- The implications that these disabilities may have for:
  - co-ordination
  - functional range of movement
  - balance
  - proprioception
  - bodily responses to physical activity
  - strength
  - endurance
  - intensity of exercise
  - flexibility and mobility.
- The types of learning difficulties that clients may have and the implications for their participation in physical activity programmes, particularly in terms of confidence, concentration and learning.
- The types of sensory impairments that clients may have and the implications for their participation in physical activity programmes.

Additionally required is knowledge from the core Level 3 Instructing Physical Activity and Exercise Knowledge requirements of units D437, D438, D439, C313, D440 and A318.

INTRODUCTION TO TRAINING
DISABLED PEOPLE

PART **ONE**

FACTS AND FIGURES

Definition of disability

Many different definitions of disability exist, often based on the purpose behind the document in which the word is used: legal, medical or personal. While some definitions impose the title on people, others allow people to choose whether to label themselves. Some individuals consider themselves to be disabled in certain circumstances but not in others, changing the label according to personal need.

Since this book makes reference to legal, medical and personal purposes at one time or another, it is helpful to use a broad definition that aligns itself well with the fitness environment.

A useful definition by Finkelstein and French (1988) is 'Disability is the loss or limitation of opportunities that prevents people who have impairments from taking part in the normal life of a community on an equal level with others due to physical or social barriers.'

The term *disability* is used throughout this book to refer to anyone who believes their life to be affected by one or more medical conditions in the long term, usually for at least one year. It includes those who were born with a medical condition and those who have acquired their condition. It includes those who are newly diagnosed with what is likely to be a long-term condition. It does not include those who have an illness or injury that is likely to impede their life for less than a year.

A more detailed investigation into the different definitions of disability is given below.

Disability statistics

It is estimated that there are anywhere between 8.6 million and 10 million disabled people in the UK. In 2000, the United Nations published research showing that the incidence of disability worldwide accounts for anywhere between 10 and 20 per cent of the population. Although these figures may seem rather varied and surprisingly high, they are in fact likely to be under-estimations. Many respondents to surveys do not classify themselves as 'disabled'. Moreover, different surveys use different definitions of disability.

While many people instantly think of wheelchair users when they think of disability (perhaps because of the symbol used to denote disability), wheelchair users actually only make up less than six per cent of the disabled population. Conditions related to obesity account for as much as 40 per cent of all disability, with recent research suggesting that by 2010 a third of the UK adult population (13 million people) will be obese.

In the UK there are estimated to be approximately:

- 10 million people with a neurological condition (Brain and Spine Foundation);
- nine million people with an arthritic condition (Arthritis Care);
- nine million deaf or hearing-impaired people (Royal National Institute for Deaf People);
- six million people with anxiety and depression (Office of National Statistics);
- two million visually impaired people (Royal National Institute for the Blind);

- 1.2 million adults with learning disabilities (Mencap);
- 400,000 wheelchair users (Spinal Injuries Association).

Cardiovascular diseases and cancer are the leading causes of early death in adults. Up to 60 per cent of wheelchair users die of cardiovascular disease. Physical activity has been shown to have a preventative effect on all of these, and has been shown to decrease disability and early death in those who already have cardiovascular disease and who introduce appropriate new activity (British Association of Cardiac Rehabilitation, 2000). The cost of physical activity in preventative healthcare may be lower than the cost of medication in curative healthcare. Physical activity also has fewer negative side-effects. The National Institute for Health and Clinical Excellence (NICE) has advised that further research is required in this area to provide more statistically reliable evidence.

The National Labour Force Survey (2000) reported there to be 6.7 million disabled adults of working age within the UK, amounting to one-fifth of the potential workforce. Research for the Joseph Rowntree Foundation (2005) found the cost of Disability Living Allowance to have increased fourfold in the past 18 years, due to an increase in the number of claimants across all age groups, not just in people over the age of 65. The assumption that disability can be associated only with people of retirement age is therefore misguided, as these figures suggest that approximately 40 per cent of the disabled population in the UK are of working age.

The financial impact of disability to the economy is staggering. For example, the cost of prescribing medications is increasing at an alarming rate. In a survey of 200 GPs across the UK published by the Mental Health Foundation in 2005, it was found that in the 12-year period from 1992 to 2003, prescriptions for antidepressants increased threefold, from 9.9 million to 27.7 million. Furthermore, the cost of these prescriptions rose by a completely staggering 2000 per cent, from £15.1 million to £395.2 million!

Despite the wealth of evidence in support of physical activity, the Health Survey for England (1998) found that only seven per cent of disabled people (compared to 31 per cent of non-disabled people) were achieving the required physical activity levels for avoidance of disease.

Only seven per cent of disabled people are sufficiently physically active for disease prevention.

Disabled people need to exercise just as much as non-disabled people and may even have a greater need if they are to maintain and/or improve their health and well-being.

According to the Chief Medical Officer (2004), adults should participate in at least 30 minutes of moderate-intensity physical activity on five or more days per week. Examples of recommended moderate-intensity everyday tasks can be seen in figure 1.1. The 30 minutes may be made up of three bouts lasting 10 minutes, or two bouts lasting 15 minutes, rather than one continuous bout. If they were to do so, adults would reduce the risk of premature death from cardiovascular disease and some cancers, and significantly reduce the risk of type II diabetes, obesity related disease and osteoporosis. Physical activity can reduce the prevalence of chronic disease by up to 50 per cent and reduce premature death by up to 30 per cent. It is no wonder that the government is trying so hard to get us all to be active!

Figure 1.1 Examples of the Chief Medical Officer's moderate activity choices

- Regular commuting on foot or by bicycle
- Regular work-related physical tasks such as delivering the post, cleaning or household decorating
- Regular household and garden activities
- Regular active recreation or social sport

These statistics hold just as true for disabled people as for non-disabled people. In fact, there are a number of factors that put some disabled people at a greater risk of diseases that result from a lack of physical activity. Many disabled people are inactive as a result of their impairment, particularly those who are unable to stand up independently. Such individuals are likely to have poor cardiovascular and digestive function, increasing the risk of life-threatening diseases such as heart disease, type II diabetes and some cancers (stomach, bowel or hormone-dependent cancers).

A review by Turk (2005) suggested that secondary conditions account for much of the ill health experienced by disabled people, more so than the primary conditions. Secondary conditions are those that are caused by a primary condition, may increase the severity of the primary condition, may be modifiable and may be preventable. Conditions that in some cases may be primary may in others be secondary. They include cardiovascular diseases (such as heart disease, diabetes or stroke), depression, obesity, osteoporosis, asthma and pain. When Guralnik et al (1993) investigated the main cause of mobility problems in older people, they found that cardiovascular disease and stroke were the main causes in men. Interestingly, for women they found it to be arthritis. Secondary conditions have been found by others (Workshop on Disability in America, 2005) not only to limit activity, but also prevent it altogether.

Depression is much more common in disabled people than in non-disabled people. A review by Kemp (2005) found that as many as 30 per cent of disabled people experience depression (compared to 10 per cent of non-disabled people). This is likely to be due to quality of life factors rather than the medical condition itself, most commonly social opportunity (Dickens and Creed, 2001). Depression has been shown to cause further secondary conditions that affect health and morbidity. For example, a survey of 10-year survival rates in people who had experienced a stroke found that those who were depressed had 30 per cent less chance of survival (Morris et al, 1993). Since many medical practitioners believe that depression is normal for disabled people, it often goes without investigation and is left untreated (Kemp et al, 2004).

Because physical activity also has a positive impact upon mental health, reducing the risk and effect of depressive illness, it has a huge role to play for those who newly acquire a disabling condition, or are living with a disabling condition that negatively affects their mental well-being. Not only does physical exercise itself help to improve mood, but benefits are also gained from the social environment inherent within most fitness facilities.

Many disabled people lose independence as their condition worsens and/or they gain secondary conditions. They may quite understandably have a negative attitude towards exercise, fearing that commencing a new exercise programme will be detrimental to their health and well-being, increasing pain and progressing disease. A poor exercise prescription, even one that follows the Chief Medical Officer's recommendations but does not take individual needs into consideration, can have just such an effect. However, the health benefits that can be gained from becoming more physically active with the correct exercise prescription may make the

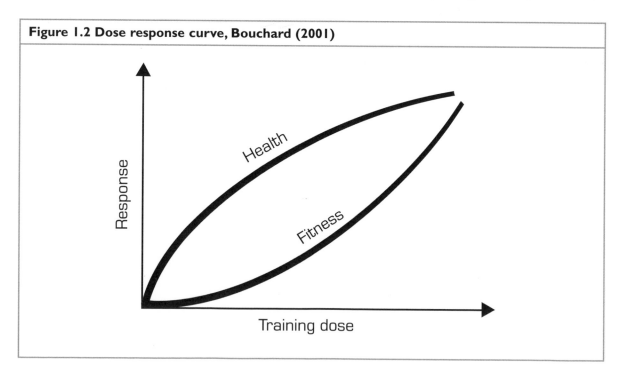

Figure 1.2 Dose response curve, Bouchard (2001)

most difference in terms of:

- Avoidance or worsening of the primary condition(s)
- Avoidance of secondary conditions
- Maintenance of independence
- Gain in independence
- Improved quality of life

For individuals for whom it would be unsafe to follow the moderate intensity of exercise that is recommended by the Chief Medical Officer (*see* fig. 1.1), intensity of exercise needs to be redefined to a more appropriate level. The dose response curve shown in figure 1.2 (Bouchard, 2001) supports this. It suggests that the greatest relative health gains are achieved when a sedentary person introduces even a minimal amount of activity into their life. As an individual becomes increasingly active, health gains do not continue to increase at the same rate. The exact level of intensity, duration and frequency that makes up the dose to achieve optimal health gains has as yet not been quantified and remains an area for further research. It should be noted that there is likely to be a different dose response curve for achieving optimal fitness gains.

Many disabled people will have been scared off exercise because they believe that a high-intensity level is necessary to achieve gains. This is not true in terms of health, though it may be the case for other gains, such as the ability to run for a bus. For such individuals, making small lifestyle changes to introduce the concept of physical activity is likely to be an effective strategy. Sometimes 'lateral thinking' may be required, as much as an education about how the medical condition, medications taken and function affect exercising ability.

If disabled people are to have anywhere near equality of opportunity to participate in the particular physical activity that is both their choice and is appropriate to their current health and fitness status, they must have access to advice. Instructors with the appropriate qualifications and increasing experience have a key role to play in providing this advice, whether the disabled person wishes to participate within a fitness facility, the great outdoors or even their own home.

Finally, it is important to recognise the social benefits that arise from exercising within a fitness facility. If the membership mix reflects everyday society, then stigmatisation of disabled people will continue to be reduced.

WHY NOW?

Legislation

In 1997 the government established the Disability Rights Task Force (DRTF), a body independent of the government, to advise on the 1997 manifesto commitment to deliver comprehensive and enforceable civil rights for disabled people. The government had recognised the lack of legislation to protect the rights of disabled people within the UK. The DRTF then set up the Disability Rights Commission (DRC) in April 2000, to champion the rights of disabled people and act as a voice for them. The DRTF and DRC were involved in advising and influencing government in the writing of the first, and subsequent, disability legislation in this country.

Before October 2004 it was permissible to refuse fitness facility entry on the grounds of disability. The Disability Discrimination Act (DDA) changed that, so that disability discrimination has now become illegal. As disabled people have started to recognise their right to attend facilities, they have met with varying degrees of success. While there is undoubtedly a need to meet this demand, there is also a need to do so in a successful manner, so that the disabled person and those they meet at the facility enjoy the experience and gain from it.

In the words of Lord Jack Ashley, a driving force behind the DDA, 'Independent living is not simply disabled people doing everything for themselves. It means ensuring that disabled people have the same freedom to choose as every other citizen and are supported in their choice in order that they may lead the lives they want to lead.'

Like most legislation, the full detail of the Act is somewhat difficult to read for those of us who are not trained to understand legal jargon! Therefore, provided here is a summary of the content that impacts upon the health and fitness industry.

The first legislation on disability in the UK was introduced in the DDA, 1995. The section on Goods, Facilities and Services, which became law in December 1996, stated the following:

1. It is illegal to refuse to serve a customer or ignore them because of a reason connected with their impairment, unless by providing the service:
   - health and safety is affected, putting the disabled person and/or others at risk;
   - the disabled person is unable to understand a contract (such as Informed Consent), although a legally appointed person could act on behalf of the disabled person;
   - it would mean no longer being able to provide the service;
   - a greater expense is involved.
2. It is illegal to provide a worse service to a disabled person.
3. It is illegal to provide a service on worse terms, such as at a higher charge.

In the same section, new laws were introduced in October 1999. Since then facilities that are open to the public have had to make reasonable adjustment, by providing extra help or making changes to the way they deliver their service. An example of this would be offering one-to-one inductions and usage supervision.

The importance of this legislation can best be seen by the changes that have occurred since its inception and by the results of test cases. To date there have been few test cases within the health and fitness industry. In one example, a local authority lost a case in which a child was refused entry to a swimming pool on the grounds that his impairment made him unsafe, even though his mother, a fully qualified swimming teacher, agreed to supervise him.

In October 2004 part three of the DDA (1995) became law. This part relates to buildings. It requires those responsible for buildings used by the public to address physical features that may act as a barrier to disabled people. This may require the removal or alteration of a physical feature, or may require providing a reasonable means of avoiding the physical feature. For example, ramps must be provided in addition to or in place of steps; signs must be larger and clearer for reading by visually impaired people; and there must be access to toilets and washing facilities. All these changes must be made on the assumption that disabled people will want to access the services; it is not acceptable to offer to make the changes as and when disabled people request them. The knowledge required to make the adjustments in advance is rather specialised and therefore companies can be hired to carry out access audits. They employ people knowledgeable about the access needs of disabled people, about building regulations, and also about the fitness industry.

In 2005 an amendment and extension to the DDA was passed. This came into force in December 2006 and there are two parts relevant to the health and fitness industry:

- Private clubs of fewer than 25 members are no longer legally able to keep disabled people excluded due to disability.
- Disability Equality Duty requires public bodies to promote equal opportunities for disabled people.

The Disability Rights Commission (DRC) has 10 'priorities for change', the first of which has influenced the new Disability Equality Duty. The DRC recognised that, while disabled people make up 20 per cent of the population, only six per cent of disabled people are involved in volunteering. This tends to reinforce the characterisation of disabled people as beneficiaries rather than contributors to their community. Disability Equality Duty is set to change this, as local authorities must promote participation by disabled people in public life, promote positive attitudes towards disabled people and actively involve disabled people in the development of policy and plans.

The UK government has come a long way in its thinking in the last 10 years, so much so that it is now working to promote the United Nations International Convention on Disability Rights. This will be legally binding in any country that ratifies it, but will also put pressure on those countries whose disability rights need improving.

Government policy and guidelines for physical activity

In 1996 the government issued a Strategy Statement on Physical Activity in which it promoted a policy advising that a minimum of 30 minutes of moderate-intensity physical activity should be completed on at least five days per week. For many disabled people this recommendation is just not feasible, often because the level of activity would worsen their condition or in some cases could be fatal. However, these guidelines are still being promoted to the British population by the National Institute for Health and Clinical Excellence (NICE).

The government has recognised that

inequalities exist in access to healthy choices. The Department of Health's white paper, *Choosing Health: Making healthy choices easier* (2004), sets out a strategy for improving opportunities by tailoring them 'to the realities of individual lives'. The realities for many disabled people mean that conventional exercise choices may not be appropriate. It goes on to state that increasing activity levels would positively impact upon the prevention and management of a large number of diseases, and it established three goals:

- For health professionals to increase the provision of lifestyle advice to patients, particularly on physical activity.
- For the development of support systems within the community healthcare system to achieve sustainable behavioural change.
- For NHS providers and primary care trusts (PCTs) to work closely with local government, private and voluntary sectors to create access to opportunities for physical activity.

A Scottish Executive document, *Delivering for Health: Building a health service fit for the future* (2005), summarised key strategies for the future as needing to be preventative. The cost of conventional 'cure' treatments is creating an impossible financial strain. Anticipatory healthcare includes the need to increase support for self-care of long term conditions and to do things 'with' instead of 'to' people. It noted that healthcare interventions are more successful if they offer opportunities for medical professionals to engage with their patients, involve their patients and empower their patients. Clearly, physical activity fits into a self-care plan and the fitness environment offers opportunities for involvement and empowerment.

Opportunities for disabled people to participate in exercise are limited when compared to the opportunities that exist for non-disabled people. The Health Education Authority's *Active for Life* campaign (1998) identified this neglect while also acknowledging that 'disabled people represent a significant proportion of the population'.

Sport England, in *Everyday Sport* (2005), a project aiming to bring physical activity into people's lives, identified disabled people as a target group, due to the barriers to exercise they face. The nature of these barriers means that this group needs targeted guidance and support when attempting to access physical activity, whether it be conventional sport, the gym, or home-based changes to daily activity levels.

These ideas are backed by European directives, which classify disabled people as a group requiring targeted assistance in its access to leisure opportunities.

Considering the number of health promotion projects that abound in most communities these days, those effectively targeting disabled people are still few and far between. As yet, only one programme, the Inclusive Fitness Initiative, has managed to effectively target and increase the activity levels of disabled people on a large scale (*see* pages 13–4).

Changes in population demographics

For some years now we have been living within an increasingly ageing population. With advances in medical science and a greater investment by people in their health, people are living for longer. This decline in early morbidity and mortality has been well documented and it is estimated that life expectancy will continue to grow.

Changes in health status that occur in adulthood often arise due to a lack of healthy living, including such factors as poor diet, smoking, alcohol and drug abuse and, of course, lack of physical activity. For many disabled people, the risks of further disease are heightened by their impairment, either directly, for example as a result of lack of movement in one or more body parts, or indirectly, for example through long-term use of medications that can lead to secondary diseases.

Additionally, disabled people have a smaller reserve capacity for life as they age. They may show characteristics of ageing earlier in life than others, so that at a younger chronological age they have an older physiological constitution. For example, osteoarthritis and the pain associated with it might have an early onset, and worsen earlier for a disabled person than for a non-disabled person.

Ethnicity, race and educational status have a marked impact on the prevalence of both impairments and the disability resulting from these impairments. While disability resulting from impairment seems to have been declining in those with higher levels of education and income, it has increased in those with lower levels of these (Schoeni et al, 2005).

Advances in medical science also mean that the survival rate of babies has improved. In years gone by, a baby born with severe impairment may have died at birth or a young person acquiring impairment experienced an early death. Now more premature babies survive, and those babies born with conditions that have in the past led to early death are surviving even into adulthood. The life expectancy and quality of life of many such individuals has grown and will continue to grow and improve. It is now estimated that disabled people account for almost 19 per cent of people of working age, totalling nearly 6.9 million.

This means that many people are living for longer with medical conditions that in earlier times may have led to an earlier death. People are living for longer, but they are living for longer with disabling conditions. According to the 2004 census, only 17 per cent of disabled people were born with impairment, with 70 per cent of disabled people acquiring their impairment during their working years. Since people are likely to live three years longer by 2020, these figures are likely to increase further, with even more disabled people making up the total adult population.

Changes in demographics of fitness facility users

In the 1970s to 1980s fitness facilities were predominantly frequented by people interested in body building. In the 1980s to 1990s they were predominantly used by people interested in fitness, often for sports-related gain. In the last 10 years, with the emergence of increasing evidence showing how physical activity can reduce the risk of many diseases and improve health, fitness facilities have been increasingly frequented by people interested in *wellness*, otherwise known as avoidance of disease and improved health.

There is a hope that increasing participation in fitness activities will lead to a decrease in the total number and severity of those diseases leading to disability that come about through a lack of physical activity.

In recent years the number of people wishing to participate in fitness-based activities has been aided by referral to exercise by medical professionals. With the dramatic increase in referral to exercise programmes (a 500 per cent increase in the last decade, from 157 schemes in 1994 to 816 schemes in 2004, according to the Chartered Society of Physiotherapists, 2004), there has been a proportionally greater increase in the number of people with medical conditions seeking to exercise. Go into any gym that has a referral programme to see how they affect the membership mix. The perception that only slim, fit, younger people attend gyms is immediately obvious as a myth. This then provides a new challenge to fitness instructors – how to meet the differing needs of the new audience to create safe, effective and enjoyable exercise sessions.

The Inclusive Fitness Initiative

The Inclusive Fitness Initiative (IFI) was the industry's response to the changing climate – an attempt to offer guidance and training to those working within leisure facilities who are concerned about meeting the requirements of the DDA.

Started in 2001, the IFI has received £6 million of Sport Lottery funding from Sport England to assist health and fitness facilities run by local authorities and charitable trusts become more compliant with the DDA. Since then, other sources of funding have enabled the project to expand to include privately run companies.

The IFI covers four key areas:

Inclusive fitness equipment

Through the development and publication of national standards for inclusive fitness equipment, the goal is to encourage equipment suppliers and purchasers to provide equipment that is accessible to both disabled and non-disabled people, so that everyone is able to exercise at the same time, using the same equipment. Equipment is tested and accredited using qualitative and quantitative feedback from a panel of specialists and testers with a range of different impairments. This feedback is given to the research and development departments of equipment suppliers. The resulting development of new equipment has raised the quality of fitness equipment and helped to solve the challenges that have previously been too much for the suppliers to overcome on their own.

Staff training

Two types of training are available. The first targets all front-of-house staff, while the second targets fitness instructors. The goal is to ensure that disabled people visiting a fitness facility will be treated with the high level of customer care they deserve.

Inclusive marketing strategies

While the first two key areas aim to cater for the needs of disabled people who attend the facility, this third area aims to communicate the facility's existence, promoting the opportunities that it offers, as for many years disabled people have been turned away from facilities. It is pointless marketing only within the facility. It is only by going out to sell the new service that perception is likely to change and disabled people can be marketed to effectively. 'Inclusive Activators' are employed to go outside the facility and work with the local community.

Inclusive development

The Fit for Inclusion service provides ongoing support and advice, including facility access audits, service and communication audits, and further tailored training.

IFI monitoring statistics are, as always, limited by the definition of disability used. In this case, people must self-declare and are not included if they choose not to declare themselves. The following statistics, as impressive as they may be, are known to undervalue the whole project. Monitoring of the project has shown that disabled people can enjoy exercising alongside their non-disabled friends and relatives. The pilot project in 2004 generated 30,000 new visits to fitness facilities by disabled people. It also showed disabled people to be a loyal market that responds well to good customer service, with 95 per cent of users stating they would continue to use the facility and 92 per cent saying they would recommend the facility to others. Since then, in a 12-month period, there were 250,000 visits by disabled people and 15,000 new inductions. Monitoring is ongoing, but current statistics show that disabled people make up seven per of all visits and 12 per cent of new users within IFI sites. Disabled people seem to attend more frequently than non-disabled people, making 2.3 visits per week.

To encourage the inclusion of private facilities and continue the good work started by the 180 sites originally on board, the IFI Mark was launched in April 2006. Supported by all the main organisations active within the fitness industry, including the Fitness Industry Association (FIA), Institute of Sport and Recreation Managers (ISRM), Institute of Leisure and Recreation Management (ILAM), Register of Exercise Professionals (REPs) and Skills Active, the Mark offers three levels of accreditation – Provisional, Registered, and Excellent – to be renewed on a biannual basis. All levels include:

- A facility access audit (new sites only)
- Inclusive equipment
- Staff training
- Marketing solutions
- Guidance on policies and procedures
- Monitoring of usage

2012 Paralympics

In 2012, not only will the Olympics come to London, but so will the Paralympics (the term meaning parallel to the Olympics). Sport England, the organisation whose role is to ensure there are opportunities for people to participate in sport and physical activity at whatever level they wish, seeks to encourage participation especially by those who are believed currently to be under-represented. Disabled people are one of their target groups, so much so that for some years now every governing body of sport has had to include within their business plans specific ideas for the development of participation by disabled people.

It is hoped that, by increasing opportunities for participation, there will be an increase in the number of people who choose to participate within sport at the highest, elite level. Training facilities must be available for elite disabled and non-disabled athletes alike. Great Britain wants to continue to hold its high position on the Paralympics medal table, second only to Australia in Sydney 2000.

Business and finance

Fitness facility managers are always interested in attracting new members, yet they know they have been trying to attract new clients from the same group of people: from those who are already members of a competitor facility. It is a highly competitive market-place. The average city-dwelling adult living in the UK has a vast choice of fitness options from which to choose. From personal training to group exercise, from basic facilities to plush designer facilities, choice has never been greater.

Disabled people offer a completely new market segment. With a little encouragement, the IFI has shown that disabled people can value the fitness experience. Although choice is currently more limited for disabled people than it is for non-disabled people, and therefore they are likely to be more loyal due to this lack of choice, disabled people are able to bring new money into the industry. Word-of-mouth is said to be the best form of advertising, and disabled people are known to successfully introduce friends and family who had not previously considered themselves suitable for the fitness experience. The success of the new business provided by disabled people has meant that the IFI has seen 50 per cent of its Inclusive Activators retained by their sites once the funding for these positions has ended.

Disabled people can be considered to be a valuable market. Marketing directly to disabled people and attracting this segment makes undeniable financial and business sense.

RISK ASSESSMENT

4

Risk assessment is necessary to ensure your safety and that of your clients before you start working together. By identifying potential hazards or dangers, and assessing the risk of them causing harm, you will be able to put into place an action plan to minimise danger.

> Hazard × Risk = Danger
> (Harm) (Likelihood)

The Health and Safety Executive (HSE, 2003) has a five-step risk assessment process, as shown in table 1.1.

Traditional risk stratification tools, such as that promoted by the American College of Sports Medicine (within the ACSM's *Guidelines for Exercise Testing and Prescription*, 2005), are based around cardiac risk factors. For the purposes of working with disabled people, clients are considered to be at low, medium or high risk, as follows:

- **Low risk**: normal heart function; free from medications that may negatively impact upon exercise; able to exercise independently within one to three sessions apart from language interpreter/some equipment set-up.
- **Medium risk**: normal heart function; taking medication(s) that may negatively impact upon exercise; requires assistance with exercising from one other person, for example gym instructor or carer.
- **High risk**: abnormal heart function; requires assistance with exercising from more than one other person; requires advanced life

Table 1.1	The HSE five-step risk assessment process
Step 1	Identify hazards or dangers Concentrate on significant hazards Ask other people involved in the activity Use own knowledge and experience
Step 2	Identify who might be harmed and how e.g. exercise professional, clients, carers
Step 3	Assess the risk: Are existing precautions adequate? What other precautions could be put into place? Who will put these precautions in place and by when?
Step 4	Record your findings
Step 5	Review the assessment periodically and revise precautions as required

Adapted from *Five steps to risk assessment*, HSE (2003)

support to be available; risk to self and/or others when in an open gym environment.

This book focuses on working with low- to medium-risk disabled people.

Disabled people who fall within a high-risk category are still likely to benefit from exercising, but not within facilities open to the general community. Such individuals are recommended to exercise within facilities where there is a mix of one or more of the following: close medical supervision; close behaviour monitoring; one-to-one supervision.

As part of a risk assessment, it is important to ensure you are appropriately trained and qualified to work with any client, disabled or otherwise.

QUALIFICATIONS

5

There are now many opportunities for instructors who wish to further their careers and develop specialist skills, especially with the success of exercise referral schemes. The qualifications framework has developed in line with this diversification to ensure instructors have the knowledge and skills required for safety and effectiveness in their work. It can be difficult to keep up with the changes in requirements, especially as there have been so many changes in the last 10 years.

The Register of Exercise Professionals (REPs) is keen to simplify the framework in order to assist instructors and the general public in understanding the qualifications.

REPs levels work in line with National/Scottish Vocational Qualification levels; currently from level one to level four. Any instructor wanting to work independently (without direct supervision) with disabled people should be registered at level three or above, with appropriate practical qualifications for the type of exercise to be performed, for example gym-based or studio-based. They should have the knowledge and skills to plan, conduct and review programmes that address the needs of disabled clients, as set out in N/SVQ Unit D442 (*see* page viii).

SUMMARY

6

There are a substantial number of disabled people living in society and, as people age, there is an increasing likelihood of acquiring a disabling medical condition. Many disabled people have a smaller reserve capacity for life and experience earlier signs of ageing.

Physical activity is an effective form of preventative medicine. It has an important role in preventing people from acquiring disabling medical conditions, preventing the incidence of further medical conditions and improving quality of life.

The current climate has created an opportunity for facilities and instructors to gain support in developing meaningful access to fitness for disabled people. Disabled people, as with all members of society, are entitled to enjoy the benefit of choice when starting a fitness regime and will gain equally, if not more, from increasing physical activity levels.

Disabled people provide a relatively untapped market segment. It makes just as much financial sense as social sense to encourage their participation. Good business people will realise that they cannot afford not to work with disabled people.

THE BACKGROUND

PART **TWO**

INTRODUCTION TO DISABILITY THEORY

7

Background theory is important to help understand our thoughts and feelings surrounding the whole subject of disability. Our thoughts and feelings will influence our values and will have a dramatic effect on the working relationships we create with disabled people, both those who are complete novices and those who are experienced exercisers. A greater understanding and depth of knowledge will influence perceptions and enhance working relationships.

In this part of the book you will find information about the barriers to participation in fitness activities that may be experienced by some disabled people and about how you may be able to minimise these barriers. There is also information about how to carry out research, so that you can become better informed and the advice you give to your clients can be based on any evidence that exists.

Views on Disability

This may be the first time that you have started to consider your own thoughts and views about disabled people. If you have not come into contact with many disabled people in the past, you may not have needed to think about your views. You may even find it difficult to decide exactly what your views are. No doubt you will have some views, consciously or unconsciously, based upon any images you may have seen in magazines or on television, and on encounters, however brief, with disabled people.

Some of the information that follows may challenge long-held perceptions and thoughts. Please do not be put off if the information does not instantly sit comfortably with you. Ensure you read the whole story, not just the opening paragraphs, before considering how it relates to your views. Persevere and consider discussing your impressions with colleagues and friends.

Approaches to disability

There are four approaches to disability that can be useful in helping to form and understand appropriate attitudes when working with disabled people.

The four approaches are:

1 Medical
2 Charitable
3 Social
4 Functional

These are summarised in table 2.1.

If fitness professionals were to work to the medical approach, they would be working alongside medical professionals to use fitness sessions as a means to a cure. Unless medically trained, this is highly inappropriate for fitness professionals and is unhelpful in enabling the disabled person to play a part in the success of their fitness experience.

If fitness professionals were to work to the charity approach, they would be encouraged to have a sympathetic rather than empathetic approach. Feeling sorry for someone to the extent that the disabled person is encouraged to be dependent on others is very different from attempting to acknowledge the individual's own

Table 2.1	Approaches to Disability		
Medical	*Charity*	*Social*	*Functional*
Owned by individual	Owned by individual	Owned by society	Owned by society
Not preventable	Not preventable	Preventable (even if *impairment* is not)	Preventable
Solution is to find a medical cure	Solution is to provide for disabled people in terms of charitable donation and support	Solution is to eliminate discrimination by removing barriers	Solution is to create inclusive opportunities

distinct set of circumstances, enabling assistance according to their own terms. Adopting the charity approach would see facilities being encouraged to offer free or discounted activity to all disabled people, not as a means of attracting them, but due to their 'tragic' circumstances. While it is true that many disabled people have a low income, there are those who do not who will be made to feel lesser citizens by this approach.

Fitness professionals who work to the social approach often find it helps to create a positive environment for both the disabled person and themselves because it encourages working 'with' rather than 'for'.

The functional approach is a relatively new concept, but is perhaps the most useful within the fitness environment. It states that it is a loss of function, resulting from a variety of factors, which causes the individual to face barriers to daily life. It asks the instructor to broadly examine the movement and/or comprehension of the disabled person. This can be achieved through discussion supported by targeted fitness testing, otherwise known as pre-exercise assessment (*see* pages 61–5). It then helps the instructor to develop a programme that develops functional fitness: that's to say, fitness for everyday life.

The functional approach is now preferred by the World Health Organisation (WHO). In 2001 WHO published its International Classification of Functioning, Disability and Health (ICF), in which for the first time it discussed the role of the environment, this being those factors outside of the individual, commonly known as extrinsic factors. The ICF refers to intrinsic factors as 'personal factors'. The ICF model of disability is shown in figure 2.1. Whiteneck (2005) has suggested that a future model could replace 'health condition' with 'quality of life', as health is only one factor in the overall quality of life of an individual.

This functional definition of disability is further reinforced by the American Institute of Medicine's definition, which defines it as 'a gap between a person's capabilities and the demands of the environment' (American Institute of Medicine, 1991). A more recent report, *Healthy People 2010*, a statement of national health objectives within the United States (United States Department of Health and Human Services, 2000), underlined the existence of extrinsic factors, citing these as being a contributor to the low provision of health promotion services for disabled people.

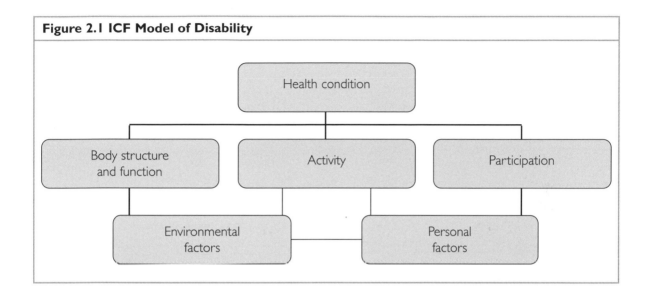

Figure 2.1 ICF Model of Disability

Barriers to participation

Disabled people face many barriers to active living and participation in fitness.

WHO (2001) defines activity and participation as follows:

- **Activity**: the execution of a task or action by an individual, not necessarily involving others (for example, washing, dressing or eating)
- **Participation**: involvement in a life situation, operating at the societal level (for example, employment in a job, or looking after the family).

There is evidence to show that severity of impairment affects activity. In other words, people with severe impairment are less likely to maintain independence in daily life. The overriding factor for participation has been found to be quality of life (Whiteneck et al, 1987 and Dijkers, 1997) rather than impairment. People who perceive they have a low quality of life are less likely to participate.

According to the Department of Health (2000), physical inactivity is associated with low social class, low income and low educational attainment. Consider a disabled person who has all of these factors against them! Having some knowledge about the factors or barriers that affect the quality of life of disabled people can enable a greater empathy or even a greater opportunity to assist in their removal. While some barriers are obviously intrinsic (pain) or extrinsic (education; finance; environment and transport; friends, family and carers), others are a mix of the two (language and communication; culture and religion; perception and attitude).

Language and communication

For many people, the fear of saying the wrong thing prevents them from interacting with disabled people. While there may be some disabled people who are interested in political correctness and are easily offended by use of

Table 2.2	Correct and incorrect language use	
Positive	**Inappropriate**	**Reason**
Disabled people	the disabled	Does not assume responsibility or ownership of disability
people with disabilities	the disabled	Places people first, but less favoured as assumes responsibility or ownership of disability
disabled people	the handicapped	Derived from 'cap in hand', or begging, suggesting that disabled people require charitable support to exist
has	suffers from	Emotive. Only each disabled person has the right to say if they suffer.
has	victim of	Again rather emotive. A victim is usually perceived to be one who has been made to suffer.
had a stroke	stroke victim	As above
person with learning disability/learning-disabled person	mentally handicapped/retarded	As above
hearing-impaired person	dumb	Playground language
person with cerebral palsy	spastic	Playground language unless used within a medical context

the wrong terms, there are others who consider politeness of attitude to be more important, and even others who do not care about language at all. It takes all sorts!

On most occasions there is no need to make use of language around disability because a person will obviously be referred to by their name. However, it is important to consider use of language for such instances as when liaising with other professionals about an individual or when advertising an activity targeted at disabled people. The most important thing is to ensure that, whatever language is used, it does not cause offence.

Table 2.2 provides a guide to positive language, inappropriate language it replaces and also the reason for the choices.

> ### Top tips for removing barriers
>
> Never let fear of using the wrong language stop you working with disabled people.

Education

Over the past 10 years there has been a change in the way disabled people experience education. While there are some 'special schools' still in existence, many disabled children now receive mainstream schooling with additional support.

Special schools are either impairment-specific (for example, for blind children) or generalised. They offer a high level of personal care and often seek to enrich life for those children with more severe impairments. They are still offered for those children who may be a risk to themselves or others within a mainstream school.

At mainstream schools, children may attend a specialised unit that offers some separate and some integrated lessons, or they may attend all lessons with non-disabled peers with additional teaching assistance where required.

The pros and cons of the different educational systems are a political minefield that shall not be discussed here. However, the pros and cons for each individual will influence their formative years and so will also influence the development of such factors as confidence, self-esteem, work ethic and capability in everyday life.

They will also influence access to meaningful physical education (PE). You will know for yourself how your earliest memories of PE lessons have influenced your views on sport ever since. The inception of the National Curriculum and Special Education Needs Act has meant that it is no longer acceptable for PE to be omitted from the curriculum offered to disabled children, or for disabled children to be made to sit and watch their non-disabled peers. However, some teachers and some schools are better than others at offering meaningful PE in which there is inclusive activity, and skills are progressed.

> ### Top tips for removing barriers
>
> The fitness environment feels very different to the school sports environment.
>
> Help newcomers to make choices about the type of exercise they would like to do by giving different options.

Finance

Many disabled people live on or near the poverty line and therefore cannot afford the expense of leisure activities, even if they have a health benefit. By contrast, there are some disabled people who are extremely wealthy and who are very able to afford to pay for the fitness experience. The Department for Work and Pensions estimates that disabled people spend £80 billion per year.

The cost of using fitness facilities can be higher for disabled people, who have to pay additional amounts for transport, carers and so on. Most fitness facilities require people to take out a membership. All-inclusive one-off memberships may not make financial sense for disabled people who are unable to predict or maintain frequency of visits. 'Pay and play' memberships, which allow payment at each visit, are much more suitable. As ever, this is all about making membership systems customer-centred rather than company-centred.

Facilities often have a policy relating to the type of clothing that should be worn while exercising. Trainers and workout wear can be expensive. As long as the clothing worn does not cause a danger to the person wearing it or to others, and does not cause offence, it should be acceptable.

Top tips for removing barriers

- Offer different types of memberships – 'pay as you go' and all-inclusive.
- Consider offering discounted usage to carers.
- Permit the wearing of everyday clothing as well as fitness clothing within your facilities.

Environment and transport

For many individuals, environment and transport can provide the greatest perceived barrier. Exercising within the home environment instantly avoids these barriers. However, disabled people will rightly want the choice of where to exercise and may want to gain access to the knowledge, skill and motivational opportunities available within a fitness facility.

There is a plan to have all public transport accessible to disabled people by 2017. Around the country, various schemes are currently available to assist disabled people with transport.

An increasing number of mobility buses are available on the public transport network, although these can run at limited, inconvenient times. Consideration then needs to be given to the distance to be travelled between the bus stop and the fitness facility.

Dial-a-ride is a national service, though it operates with regional variations. An annual membership fee is usually charged for the provision of a door-to-door service by an accessible bus. The driver of the bus will have received disability equality training and will be trained to assist with getting on and off the bus. The drawback of this service is its popularity, causing challenges with time-keeping.

In some parts of the country, travel assistance schemes operate to offer help with accessing the local public transport. For example, in London a 'buddy' can be booked for a series of travel sessions, with the goal being to increase confidence and skills for independent travel in the future.

For those who drive, the 'Motability' scheme provides financial support for the purchase and adaptation of a suitable car. Parking bays for disabled people should be clearly marked and provided near to the entrance of the facility. These are usually wider than other parking bays to allow space for the car door to fully open and for transfer to and from a wheelchair.

The route between the car park and facility should be clearly marked and consideration given to lighting and to maintaining a level or ramped surface.

Top tips for removing barriers

Carry out a transport survey and include a transport map in your marketing material. Include information on public transport (bus routes, bus stops and train stations), assisted transport, car parking, walking paths and lighting.

Culture and religion

The teachings of some cultures and religions may impact upon the exercise choices available. For example, some Asian religions and some branches of Judaism do not permit men and women to exercise together, with some only allowing women to exercise in a closed area that cannot be overlooked by men. This can make it even more difficult for disabled people to find a suitable facility.

Some religions do not allow the carrying of money and/or participation in sporting activities on holy days. Consider if the only access to your specialist advice was on a Sunday; disabled people coming from some branches of Christianity would be prevented from gaining access to you. A colleague of mine once set up an open sports session on a Friday evening, forgetting that the area was populated by lots of Jewish people for whom this is the start of the Sabbath. He found the session much more successful once it was changed to a Wednesday evening!

Top tips for removing barriers

- Find out about the cultural and religious mix of the local population. Use this information when preparing the fitness class timetable.
- Keep an updated log of single-gender exercise opportunities in your facility and other facilities within your locality.
- Offer advice on home exercise to complement opportunities at your facility.

Friends, family and carers

Friends and family can make all the difference to the success or failure of a new exercise regime. Many disabled people will be reliant on their friends and family for more than just moral support. They may require assistance with transport, communication or administration of a Pre-Activity Readiness Questionnaire (PAR-Q).

While some disabled facility users will be able to travel and use a fitness facility independently, others will be dependent on friends, family or care workers to support them. For those disabled people who do not have a legal age of consent, usually set at 18 years, a legal advocate will need to be present when the PAR-Q is administered.

While many carers provide a wonderful source of support and inspiration, others have no interest in exercise and create obstacles through their negative attitudes. This can be especially noticeable in the case of disabled people who require support in everyday life and are reliant on others for planning their daily activities. It can be very difficult to increase activity levels if carers do not follow the guidance given by fitness instructors.

More supportive carers will be keen to become involved in assisting with the success of the disabled person's exercising experience.

With a small amount of training, they can free up the time of the instructor to spend with others. However, carers who are less keen can create a negative experience for all. In such cases, if it is possible to ask the carer to provide any necessary personal assistance outside of the exercising environment, but not get involved within the exercising environment, this can lead to greater success.

> **Top tips for removing barriers**
>
> - Advise anyone who does not have legal consent to attend their first session with a legal advocate.
> - Give carers a role to play, either including them in the fitness session or asking them to return at a set time after the session has ended.

Pain

If you have ever had times when you have experienced pain, you will also have experienced how the pain affected your motivation as well as your ability to perform everyday tasks and to participate in life. Not only does pain cause fatigue, but the fear of making it worse leads to sedentary behaviour. Leveille et al (1999) unsurprisingly found that pain significantly impacted upon the ability to perform various tasks of everyday life, making the tasks more difficult to perform. However, perhaps surprisingly, they also found that pain did not significantly relate to whether people could or could not perform the tasks at all. Pain is closely linked to perception.

> **Top tips for removing barriers**
>
> - Advise newcomers that physical activity has been shown to help in the management of pain caused by most medical conditions.
> - Advise newcomers that they are never going to be forced to do an exercise, but will be consulted before being advised.

Perception and attitude

Many people who are currently not members of fitness facilities believe that exercise is not for them, either because exercise would be too hard or because facilities are unsuitable for their needs. The perception that exercise must be painful and hard in order to be effective is a myth perpetuated by the media and forced home in reality television programmes. The view that facilities are frequented by highly fit individuals is another myth only further reinforced by adverts in the media.

For those who have not visited fitness facilities within the last 10 years, a belief that gyms are for body-builders or disciples of Jane Fonda may still be putting them off.

Disabled people face a further barrier with the belief that they will be met by unhelpful staff and will require specialist exercise equipment. In the case of disabled people who, before the DDA was in existence, were turned away from facilities, it may be very difficult to convince them those times have changed. It was not long ago that a receptionist would only allow entry to the disabled swimming club, even though the individual wanted to go to the gym!

Not only do perceptions held by disabled people create barriers for them, but so too do the perceptions of those around them, including those working within the facilities. Their perceptions are equally hard to change.

The IFI training aimed at all front-of-house staff has been shown to be extremely important in addressing this. Disabled people meeting receptionists or instructors with a negative attitude will not return to the facility for fear of being made to stand out or being made to feel a fool.

Perceptions are very difficult to break. People who have held their perceptions for many years will *know* them to be true, regardless of new information gained or influences otherwise!

Top tips for removing barriers

- Introduce disabled people to other disabled facility users as soon as possible.
- Encourage people to attend with their friends and/or family.
- Try to avoid using jargon and instead use phrases from people's everyday lives that help them to associate with exercise.
- Ensure every visit has a positive outcome, however small this may seem.

BEHAVIOURAL AND MOTIVATIONAL THEORY

8

Introduction

Every member of society has a responsibility to lead a healthy lifestyle, including participating in physical activity. The difficulty comes in providing the support and motivational techniques required to assist each individual to follow through with what they realise they should be doing.

Many people believe that their local leisure facilities are unsuitable for their needs. Many will believe that fitness is not for them. They will believe this to the extent that they *know* it to be true. Disabled people's beliefs are no different from those of non-disabled people in this area, though the reasons for their beliefs may come from different origins.

The DDA has provided a new opportunity for disabled people to become more active. Leisure providers must offer their services to disabled people or risk facing legal action. As a result, those who were not taking steps to make their facilities accessible have recently improved opportunities for disabled people. The discrimination is lessening; yet helping disabled people to take the plunge and try joining a fitness facility may involve a psychological battle. The discrimination existed for many years, so it may take a long time to convince disabled people that times have changed. An understanding of the psychological barriers put up by disabled people is very helpful when trying to break down those barriers.

To achieve a successful relationship with a person who is yet to be convinced that participating in exercise will be a positive experience, it is essential for trust to be developed. Themes from the field of psychology help in understanding why each disabled person behaves in a different way, how to go about addressing any negative behaviour and how to assist each person with an individualised approach to creating a long-term physical activity strategy.

People with the same impairments may be aggressive or friendly, shy or extrovert, confident or nervous. Clearly, although these individuals may have the same physical needs, their psychological needs differ greatly. Every person is an individual, with a distinct set of physical characteristics and personality traits. Each individual therefore should be dealt with in an individualised manner, from the manner of communication you adopt through to the exercise programming.

Various models and theories from the field of psychology have been used to help understand why people do or do not choose to do things in life and, most importantly, what the fitness industry can do to increase the chances of people choosing fitness activities. Some of these ideas from psychology are presented below to assist in appreciating why people behave as they do and what you can do to help influence negative attitudes and behaviour towards fitness.

'Truth'

The social cognitive model (Bandura, 1960s) provides a useful tool for understanding the internal influences on an individual's motivation to take part in regular physical activity. The model basically says, 'I act as I think I am'. It shows how people will always act in a way that is true to themselves. As such, it helps in the understanding of how each individual's 'truth' is arrived at and how that 'truth' is different according to their past experiences. 'Truth' is given in inverted commas to suggest that the truth may not be factually true, but actually a personalised account, or a perception.

A person's 'truth' may in fact be far from the truth. If an individual has held a thought for many years, it will be very difficult for them to accept that in fact it is not true. They may put up a resistance to change, especially if they are unsure whether the consequences will be beneficial. They may have decided that the risks far outweigh any potential benefits.

People's 'truths' not only affect how they behave outwardly, but also how they think inwardly. Everyone has a continuing chatter going on in their head, known as 'self-talk', telling them how they feel about everything that is going on in their life. The 'creative subconscious' is then responsible for making sure they act in accordance with who they believe they are. While some people have a tendency to be positive in their self-talk, others can be very negative. For example, when going for an interview, one interviewee could have a self-talk saying, 'There's going to be someone there better than me; I'm not sure I'll be the best person for the job,' while another may have a self-talk saying, 'I'm going to do brilliantly today. They'll all like the fact that I'm well qualified.' Which of these people do you think would be more likely to get the job?

Consider a disabled person who at school was not able to enjoy PE. No doubt they built up negative perceptions around exercise, as is fairly typical for many non-disabled people too! Throughout their adult life, this disabled person is then likely to only consciously notice negative information about exercise, in order to back up their original thinking. They will 'know' that exercise is unsafe for them. They are not interested in hearing that, while certain types of exercise may be unsafe, others may not only be safe but even good for them! They are unable to give even a moment's thought to something that is at odds with their 'truth'.

Perception

People are constantly taking in information from their surroundings to influence their thinking. They do this not only consciously, but also unconsciously. Most of the information from the environment is filtered out by a part of the brain known as the reticular activating system. If it were not for the reticular activating system, we would all be so overloaded with information that we would be unable to get on with life! People will only take notice of what is relevant to them, either because it has something positive to offer or is dangerous. Each person's perception of what is of interest, or even what is dangerous, differs as a direct result of all their past experiences and their current list of wants.

Case study

I used to have a business offering exercise classes in a venue on a busy high street. A year after it began, I was still getting enquiries from people who had walked past every day but only just noticed the advertising board. They were convinced the business was new and found it hard to believe they could have walked past without noticing it. They would comment what an amazing coincidence it was that they should have noticed just as they were starting to think about going to classes.

This was no coincidence. Their mind was no longer filtering out the advertising board because it was now relevant. This is also why, in a crowded room, you will usually hear your name being mentioned even when someone is saying it from the other side of the room. You may not have heard any of the previous conversation but this is important to you and you will notice it – after all it could be a threat to you! Consider a wild animal that should be scared of humans, but as a result of learning that human contact often means food, becomes tame. Humans are no different from other animals in redefining danger according to past, learned experience.

Behaviour

Neuro-linguistic programming (NLP, Grinder and Bandler, 1970s) shows the connection between the mind (neuro), language (linguistic) and purposeful actions or behaviours (programming). According to NLP, every thought has a physical response, and every physical action has an associated thought. It also introduces the idea that people will only behave in ways that are true to themselves and not in conflict with their inner self.

NLP suggests that all actions are useful, with the definition of usefulness depending on each individual's personal set of beliefs. Therefore, if the instructor meets a group of disabled people who have consistently received the message that gyms are not appropriate for them, the disabled people are unlikely to believe there is any gain to be had from attending a gym and the instructor will have a battle to get any members of that group willingly to attend. If the instructor listens carefully, they will be able to use this information to their advantage, drawing on it as a starting point when explaining how the facility and the staff within it will meet the needs of the group.

Since it is clear that our thoughts and behaviours are linked, there is an opportunity for the physical benefits of exercise to impact positively upon thoughts. Research into exercise and mood has shown repeatedly that exercise can improve mood and is now recommended as a first line of therapy (before medication) for some forms of depression. If a disabled person has low self-esteem, it is likely that this will express itself in many ways: in negative self-talk, slouched posture and either an aggressive or apathetic manner. Physical activity in a supportive environment may not only affect the person's fitness levels, but also their self-talk, their posture and their overall demeanour. I once had a client who suddenly decided that the exercise had given her so much confidence that she was now ready to find a job! Exercise can be truly life-changing.

Thinking point

Think back to the earlier example of two people going to a job interview, one having negative self-talk and the other having positive self-talk. When you first thought about these two individuals, what pictures of them did you see in your mind? It is likely that while the first image was of someone who looked tired and pale, with a slouched posture, the second image was of someone who was standing upright, looking proud and dressed elegantly. There is no doubt that self-talk affects self-image (as shown in fig.2.2). What other perceptions did you have about these people? With which one of these people would you most like to associate? Which one most closely reflects you?

People tend to gain the confidence and motivation to do things by observing others who are, like themselves, successfully doing those very things. It is partly due to the lack of

mass-media images showing different people doing fitness activities that so many disabled people do not perceive the fitness environment to be for them. Most of these images show young or middle-aged muscular men and toned women exercising in lycra. Sport England accepts that mass-media images have not helped to attract new individuals, especially disabled people, into the fitness arena. In their document, *Understanding Participation in Sport* (2005), they note the importance of including a range of images involving different population groups successfully participating in a variety of activities.

Motivation

What motivates you to exercise? If you are in your 20s, it is unlikely to be the avoidance of disease when you get into your 60s! People often say they are going to exercise classes 'to

Figure 2.2 The self-image cycle

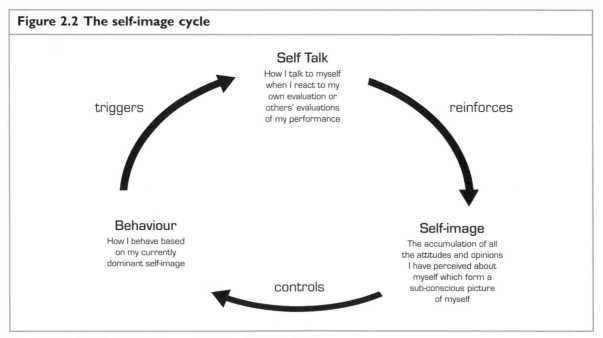

Self Talk
How I talk to myself when I react to my own evaluation or others' evaluations of my performance

triggers

reinforces

Behaviour
How I behave based on my currently dominant self-image

Self-image
The accumulation of all the attitudes and opinions I have perceived about myself which form a sub-conscious picture of myself

controls

From YMCAfit Inclusive Health, Fitness and Activity: Disability, 2005

get fit'. People have many and varied reasons for why they want to exercise and many different interpretations of the word 'fitness'.

According to behavioural theory, humans are motivated by the pursuit of rewards. These rewards could be perceived by others to be large (such as finishing first in a race), or they could be perceived by others to be small (such as attending the gym for the first time); they could be extrinsic (such as winning a medal, hearing praise), or intrinsic (such as improvements in self-belief). For many people who are new to exercise, intrinsic motivators are more powerful.

Many disabled people will have low levels of self-belief, affecting their confidence and ability to participate in every part of daily life. Fitness instructors have the opportunity to influence self-belief from the moment they meet potential new clients. The following suggestions show how this can be achieved:

- A tour of the facilities that shows other disabled people participating successfully ('If they can do it, so can I')

- Words of praise and encouragement ('My instructor says I can do it and so I believe I can too')
- Information about what can be expected to happen while exercising, both physically and mentally ('My instructor says it's normal to expect my breathing rate to go up, so I shouldn't be scared')
- The achievement of some level of success on every occasion ('I'm looking forward to coming back').

The transtheoretical model of change (Prochaska and DiClemente, 1984) helps to explain whether an individual is likely to be interested in attending regular fitness sessions and whether they are likely to adhere to exercise in the long term. The stages of the model can be seen in figure 2.3.

How each stage affects likelihood of participation and how you can work appropriately with people in the different stages is described as follows:

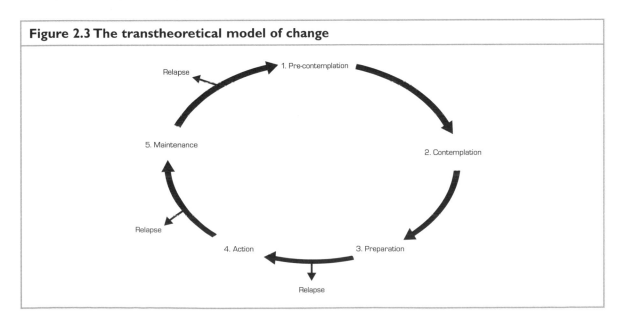

Figure 2.3 The transtheoretical model of change

1. Pre-contemplation
Relapse
5. Maintenance
2. Contemplation
Relapse
4. Action
3. Preparation
Relapse

1 Pre-contemplation

In pre-contemplation an individual will have no interest in exercise and will not notice marketing that may appear in newspapers, magazines or on billboards. They will not associate themselves with exercise in any manner whatsoever. Many disabled people will fall into this category, having undergone years of inactivity due to physical and/or psychological barriers to participation. They have either never considered exercise or are 'anti' it for a number of reasons. You are unlikely to be able to convince someone in pre-contemplation that their ideas are incorrect.

2 Contemplation

Within the general population, it is not unusual for people to spend up to six months at this stage. Disabled people are more likely to remain in this stage for years. People at this stage are open to suggestion. They require support to review and reflect on their current lifestyle and how an increase in physical activity could improve it. They require support and guidance, with provision of user-friendly facts about the type of activity that might be suitable and how they can go about accessing it. People should be given encouragement while in contemplation, but should not be pushed into moving forwards. Everyone needs to be given the time and space that is suited to them.

3 Preparation

This stage involves people taking the first steps towards becoming a regular exerciser. This is the stage when people start going to exercise classes or the gym, possibly going with a friend or family member to help motivation. It is a crucial stage and positive reward for participation is vital if there is to be any chance of a disabled participant moving to the next stage. Every session should involve reward, whether it is improvement in physical ability or simply enjoyment of the exercising environment. Would you continue to do something that was not enjoyable? Rewards for disabled people can be social, psychological and/or physical.

4 Action

The first six months are absolutely crucial, as it is during this time that relapse is most common. Reasons for continuing exercise must be made apparent. The likelihood of relapse is significantly higher with disabled people due to both intrinsic (to do with the individual) and extrinsic (to do with others) factors, including poor self-esteem, demands of personal assistants, worsening of medical conditions, or institutional arrangements.

It is vital at this stage that the disabled person has built up relationships with staff and other users at the fitness facility. The more friends there are to see, the more likely the person is to want to attend. It is also important that the disabled person can see measurable progress is being made and that this progress is related to their own personalised goals.

5 Maintenance

Disabled people who start to enjoy exercising regularly will still need reminding of the many benefits and of how achievement of their early goals has impacted on their lives. Plateauing – reaching a point where there is no more marked improvement – and boredom can rapidly lead to relapse, so re-evaluation and further goal-setting are vital. Again, relationships with others are important, especially if those others are responsible for getting the person to their exercise session.

6 Relapse

Although relapse is extremely common and is best thought of as inevitable, research from the IFI has shown that disabled people who exercise within

IFI-accredited facilities do not seem to drop out of exercise. Although nobody is currently sure why this is, it is likely to be linked to the level of friendliness and support offered by the staff at these facilities. Be aware that relapse is very common and attempt to find out what motivates each individual in order to develop strategies to deal with it before, rather than after, it happens.

Case study

An obese man, who was unable to work due to immobility, pain and depression, joined his local gym after gaining GP consent. He was very keen, evidenced by how hard he worked on every visit and his friendliness with staff. Because he was so keen to lose the weight and had nothing else to do, he attended the gym every weekday. During the first month he lost 10 pounds in weight and was pleased with this result. At first glance this seems to be the ideal scenario, of a man ready to take on exercise into the future, but . . .

Whenever gym instructors had time to spend with him he would talk almost non-stop. He revealed information in his chatter that was ignored. In his first assessment and over his first month of membership he had mentioned that this was not the first time he had tried using exercise to help him lose weight; in fact, he had tried it four times previously. Each time he found he was really keen to begin with, but after approximately three months he had lost the motivation. It all seemed like too much hard work to have to keep exercising and get sweaty everyday.

Do you think this latest attempt was likely to prove successful?

The gym instructors were missing important information being offered by their client. Early keenness seemed to lead to early fatigue; not only physical fatigue but, most importantly, mental fatigue. They should have been advising him to exercise on no more than three occasions each week and should have been limiting the intensity of each workout. Careful listening skills should have been used to constantly assess his level of motivation.

In order to make motivators work, it is helpful to fit them into a framework, best known as SMART goal setting (*see* fig. 2.4).

As you discuss your clients' goals with them, listen carefully to the words they use. Attempt to use these words when you come up with the final wording of the goal. Many clients will not use exercise jargon when they talk about their wants. Phrases like 'aerobic fitness' are often meaningless to our clients. Words such as 'I want to be able to walk to the letterbox without getting out of breath' mean exactly the same thing in reality, but they 'belong' to the individual and help association. Always try to remember that this is their exercise programme; the role of the fitness instructor is to educate and motivate. Unfortunately for our clients, we cannot do it for them!

Wherever possible, try to express SMART goals in a positive sentence. Goals surrounding weight can be expressed either as weight loss (negative), fat loss (negative), or achieving or fitting into a certain clothing size (positive). People generally like to gain things in life; our minds do not like the idea of losing things! It is no wonder that so many people fail to achieve their ideal weight!

Various research studies have shown that one of the greatest motivations for exercise is not actually associated with the exercise itself, but with the environment in which the exercise is performed. In the Sport England report, *Participation in Sport: A Systematic Review* (2005), the following were found to be the most popular reasons for participation:

- Health benefits
- Weight management
- Social interaction
- Enjoyment

Figure 2.4 SMART goal-setting

Specific State the goal in clear English, if possible using phrases spoken by the client. The nearer the goal is to their language, the more likely they are to associate with it.

Measurable State numbers (repetitions, distances, weights, ratios, percentages) to ensure that when revisited changes can be easily noted.

Agreed Negotiate with the individual. The goal is theirs, not yours. Refuse to be part of a goal that is unhealthy (for example, 'I want to lose two stone in two months'), but equally the individual has the right to refuse to be part of goals in which they have no interest (such as 'Use this new health drive as an opportunity to give up smoking').

Realistic Set goals that you know require a certain amount of effort, but that you know the client can achieve. Remember to tailor the progress appropriately for each individual.

Time-framed If the overall goal is likely to take months or years to achieve, set other short-term goals (up to six weeks). Identify what should be achieved by when.

Case study

When visiting an IFI site recently I was pleased to see a wall covered with cards that had been completed by grateful gym members. Every card was set out in the same way, with tick boxes and spaces for comments. The cards had been filled in by new members who had completed 12 weeks of attendances. Each card asked why the member was attending and whether they were along the road to achieving their goal. It all looked very impressive. But when I then read each of these cards, I was disappointed at the level of communication and the lost opportunity for insightful information.

Each card only offered a choice of five different goal options (weight loss; improved fitness; improved strength; improved flexibility; other). What was more, every card but one had weight loss as the selected goal option. Was almost every person using this facility really only interested in losing weight? Or could it be that they did not understand what improved fitness, improved strength and improved flexibility actually meant? Would it not have been better to give the individual an empty space in which to express himself or herself? How many of these members are still actively attending? I am unaware of the answer, but I bet I could hazard a guess.

Motivational interviewing

Motivational interviewing was first identified by William Miller in 1983, in relation to his work treating problem-drinkers. He defines it as: 'a directive, client-centred counselling style for eliciting behaviour-change by helping clients explore and resolve ambivalence' (Rollink and Miller, 1995).

Motivational interviewing provides an opportunity to help the client lead the way in the plan for a new exercise programme. It is pointless for the instructor to suggest things that the client has no interest in doing. There should always be a respect for each other and for the client's rights to engage or not engage in an activity.

Motivational interviewing techniques allow the client to lead the sessions; they encourage the client to be more focussed, to help work towards their own goals. It requires the fitness instructor to learn to listen and observe their client carefully, to receive feedback signals about negative thoughts that create confusion or contradiction, and positive thoughts that lead to motivation. The instructor never tells the client how they should be thinking, but asks questions to assist the client in finding answers for himself/herself. Through creating a relationship built on mutual respect, the client is assisted and supported on their own terms.

Excellent instructor communication skills are at the core of motivational interviewing.

FINDING OUT MORE

Introduction

Throughout this book, reference is made to research. Research is necessary for two reasons:

- the continuing professional development of every fitness professional;
- your safety and that of anyone you instruct.

It is essential that all your clients' medical conditions are investigated, whether primary or secondary (a condition arising as a result of another condition).

Research can be daunting, especially if it is written in scientific language and presents lots of statistical analysis. Below you will find advice on how to conduct research and how to improve knowledge on specific fitness information. Consider your style of learning and select those research formats that best suit you. Remember to then question what is presented. Not only will your investigations add detail to your current knowledge and views, they may also be at odds with them! By analysing the information, you will be surprised to find how many research studies carried out to date have been flawed in their approach. Finding out more is a journey of discovery that creates a more detailed picture and often leads to further questions.

Consider the following in your research into fitness for disabled people:

- Whether the study was scientific or non-scientific/anecdotal
- Whether study subjects were disabled people
- The size of group used – a small group may not be reflective of that population

- Whether the participants had only the one condition being investigated, or had co-existing conditions that may have influenced the results
- Whether the people with progressive medical conditions were at the same stage of the condition
- Whether everyone in the study was taking the same, different or no medications
- Whether the duration of the study was sufficient – less than 12 weeks tends to make conclusions impossible, or leads to information being missed.

Your clients are often a wonderful resource for the start of any research. They often have a very good understanding of their condition(s) and most importantly will be able to explain how they affect them. Conditions do not tend to affect everyone the same way. This is also true for many medications, with some people experiencing no side-effects and others experiencing many side-effects.

Regardless of the information given by the client, it is essential to access other means of background information. Unfortunately there is a very limited amount of published scientific research about the effect of medical conditions on physical activity. The research that does exist tends to be descriptive (comments on populations) rather than researched (results from experiments). In fact, the American College of Sports Medicine (ACSM), having recognised the lack of research and therefore lack of scientifically-based guidance for fitness professionals, sees this as an important area for them to investigate over the coming years.

Questions such as how exercise impacts upon people with specific medical conditions, both physically and psychologically, and what type of exercise at what level of intensity they should do, remain to be answered.

Other than some excellent studies on cardiovascular diseases, the few studies that have been carried out have tended to answer very specific questions, such as the effect of aerobic exercise on thermoregulation in paraplegic athletes. This is hardly useful to the majority of fitness professionals, being that we do not tend to measure thermoregulation; nor do most of our clients have the fitness of elite athletes!

Many of the current recommendations are based on research carried out on non-disabled people. For example, throughout this book reference is made to copious research proving that lack of physical activity causes disease and early death and suggesting how to engage more people in physical activity. None of this research has knowingly been carried out on disabled people (other than people with cardiovascular diseases), and so it cannot be safely assumed the same messages on levels of physical activity hold true.

Over the years, many medical professionals and people involved in rehabilitation (such as physiotherapists and occupational therapists) have anecdotally shared their successes. This had led to a certain amount of useful information becoming available for adapting general guidelines when working with people who have specific medical conditions.

Sources of information

There are many sources of research information available. They include:

- fitness industry colleagues in the same or other facilities
- referring medical professionals, including

consultants, UKs, nurses, physiotherapists, osteopaths and occupational therapists
- books and journal articles (*see* References and Further Reading on page 155)
- the internet (*see* Useful Websites on pages 157–8).

Fitness industry colleagues

As a result of personal experiences (disabled friends or family) or work-related training (previous jobs or current health-related jobs), these people are a wonderful resource of instant, user-friendly information. Not only are they able to provide information on the medical conditions, but they also have an appreciation of the context and the fitness industry. They provide an opportunity for two-way communication, enabling questions relating to the specific circumstances of an individual disabled person.

Top tips for gaining information from colleagues

I have a list of friends within the industry who I know to have experience of certain conditions. They are able to provide me with insightful information and I am able to ask questions without worrying that I will make a fool of myself.

Medical professionals

While some medical professionals are welcoming of questions, others can be difficult to access. Some have a greater understanding of the needs of the fitness professional than others. There are those who believe in the power of physical activity as an alternative or addition to medication, while there are still some who are not keen to promote physical activity and may even choose to steer their patients away from it altogether. With the growth of referral schemes and the Medical Defence Union's acknowledgement of the role of appropriately qualified Advanced Fitness Instructors, the understanding between the industries is growing. Recognising and being sensitive to our similarities and our unique differences is essential for the creation of successful working relationships.

Referring medical professionals are often keen to assist in providing a positive exercising experience for their patients. Due to their lack of experience within the fitness industry, they may not know what information is helpful, and so may provide limited information at the time of referral. However, when asked specific questions they are only too pleased to provide the answers. These answers can sometimes be delivered in a rather technical manner. Never be afraid to ask for further explanation or decoding of jargon. Remember, we have a set of jargon in our industry that they would not understand either!

Top tips for gaining information from medical professionals

While some medical professionals can be contacted by telephone or in person, others may be difficult to access in this manner. The development of standardised referral materials (emails/letters) within your workplace can prove extremely helpful.

Books and journal articles

Books and journal articles can usually be said to be current if published within the last three years, although older resources may still be valid. This is especially the case within the context of this subject, as the research into physical activity and disability is so limited. As such, any that exist should be carefully considered!

While there are very few books that provide information on how medical conditions influence exercise programming, there are many that provide information on medical conditions. These books are targeted at different audiences, from medical students to family members, and so the language they use varies enormously. Generally, the more technical ones provide the greatest scientific details. Sometimes they provide more information than is required, but becoming acquainted with medical jargon can assist when liaising with medical professionals.

Journal articles, which publish scientific research, are another useful source of information. However, they can also be full of technical information written in scientific or medical jargon. Rarely do we need to read the analysis of the statistical data, especially as it can be impossible to understand if you are not used to reading research! But the abstract, or summary, often provides de-jargonised technical information in sufficient detail to allow understanding of the key messages. If you are able to find a useful article, my advice is to read the abstract, then only continue with the remainder of the article if you want to learn more and are trained in how to read it.

Top tips for gaining information from books and journals

Use those recommended by colleagues as being written in a user-friendly manner for fitness instructors. When reading journal articles, start with the abstract.

The internet

Since the introduction of the internet into most homes and workplaces, the opportunities for research have dramatically opened up. The difficulty now is sourcing the information required from the hundreds of responses to a search question and then ensuring that any responses are from trustworthy sites. While anecdotal evidence can be interesting, the small sample size (often just the person writing the piece – that is, a sample size of one!) and sponsorship behind the article (an interested party) mean that the information may not be exactly correct or trustworthy.

Top tips for gaining information from the internet

Selecting from online journals and online disability organisations is usually worthwhile. Those that come from sites in this country ending .gov (government) or .ac (academic) are useful, as they are public organisations that carry a responsibility to only display valid, accurate information.

Top tips for carrying out research

Whichever sources of information are selected, it is important to ensure the information gathered is technically correct and provides sufficient background to the medical condition for programming and instruction purposes. While plentiful information may be found about a specific condition, it is important to prioritise it on a need-to-know basis.

RECORDING INFORMATION

10

Creating your own resources

As you carry out your research and gather information about the client, their form and functional abilities, it is important to have an organised way of recording your findings. Scraps of paper can be good initially, but if you are anything like me you will soon lose them! Have a folder or book in which to keep all your information together and consider having this available as a reference manual for everyone with whom you work. Encourage them to add to it, as and when they have gathered new information. It will soon grow to provide a user-friendly, easily accessible source of information in itself.

Pro-forma

The headings below provide a useful 10-step framework from which to work when gathering information in preparation for working with a disabled person.

1 Name of condition
2 Definition of condition – a summary description in one or two sentences
3 Main characteristics of condition – how the condition usually presents physically and psychologically
4 Effects of the condition on exercise response
5 Medications – what medications are commonly prescribed and any effects or side-effects that impact upon exercise response
6 Important rules – any definite do's or don'ts related to, and resulting from, 4 and 5, above
7 Goals of the exercise programme
8 Programming principles – considering the effect of all of the above information (points 2 to 7) on the session components and components of fitness in terms of FITTA principles (*see* page 69).
9 Teaching principles – using all of the above information (points 2 to 8), consider the effect of these on fitness instruction, including instructing each exercise and recording each exercise session.
10 Having gathered the above information, further information on the needs and wants of the specific client should be added to ensure a fully personalised exercise programme and instructional approach. For a blank pro-forma document that you can copy for your own use, please see Appendix 2 on pages 151–2.

SUMMARY

11

Everybody is an individual. Those with similar medical conditions will have different personalities and those with similar personalities will have different medical conditions. That's life!

It is important to consider your own thoughts about disabled people. Where have your perceptions come from? Do your thoughts differ for unfit disabled people compared with sporty disabled people? Do they currently, and will they in the future, either help or hinder your work? Can you open your conscious thoughts to entertain new concepts that challenge your 'truths'? Also consider the perceptions disabled people are likely to have about you. How can you help disabled people feel comfortable with you if you know that they are uncomfortable and nervous with the concept of fitness?

Ensure you use the resources that are around you when carrying out research. Give yourself the time to carry out research, using the sources of information that best suit your learning style. Keep any new information in a folder, so that you know where it is should you want to access it again in the future.

PROGRAMMING AND INSTRUCTION

PART THREE

WORKING WITH DISABLED PEOPLE

12

In this part of the book you will find practical advice on how to work safely with disabled people, from the moment they express interest in starting to exercise, through to regular supervision of an exercise programme. Clear guidance is given on how to offer a high level of duty of care throughout the programming and instruction process: when planning and programming; when instructing; and when monitoring and reviewing each subsequent session.

Figure 3.1 shows how all of these factors interrelate and demonstrates the importance of consulting with each participant to ensure they remain as the focus and at the centre of the decision-making process.

Figure 3.1 The role of the instructor

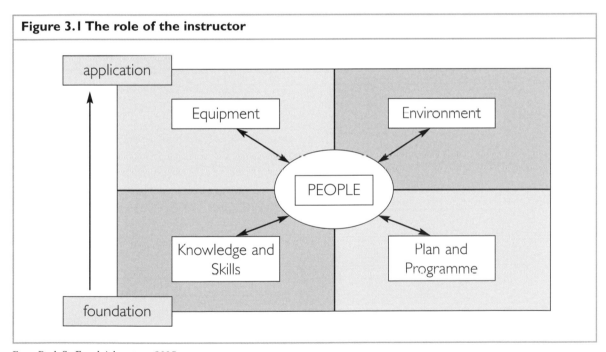

From Paul, S., Equal Adventure, 2005

PRE-ACTIVITY HEALTH AND SAFETY

13

Introduction

Before the participant commences exercise it is essential to carry out a risk assessment (*see* Chapter 4) and to gather background information about the client. Taking a little extra time at this stage can save wasted hours later and may also prevent injuries or illnesses unfolding within the exercise environment.

Duty of care

Duty of care refers to the responsibilities of the instructor and anyone else with whom the disabled person may come into contact during their visit to a fitness facility. Instructors should already be aware of the Health and Safety at Work Act (1974), which lays out the responsibilities of all staff within their workplace. It states that every employee or self-employed person must show a duty of care to themselves and other persons. In most instances the Health and Safety at Work Act can be fairly easily interpreted within the fitness environment. However, the health and fitness industry often lacks clarity in law in clearly determining the responsibilities of staff and users, making it difficult to know exactly what specific requirements there might be.

The case study below and previous findings (such as Glasgow Corporation vs. Taylor, 1922 and Haley vs. London Electricity Board, 1965) help to clarify the provisions of the law.

Case study

A court case took place in 1993 (Morrell vs. Owen), in which a sports coach was found guilty of negligence after a disabled person was injured during a sports session. The disabled person had sat in a dangerous place while activities were going on around her, and although she had repeatedly been asked to move, she had refused to do so. The judge stated that the duty of care owed to disabled participants was greater than that owed to non-disabled participants. He also said that the responsibilities of coaches working with disabled people included instructing them in safe procedures and practice for moving in and out of practice areas, and providing someone to watch over their movements.

Responsibility therefore does not start and end simply with safe instruction of the actual activity by the instructor. It also includes ensuring safety from the time the disabled person enters the facility to the time they leave. While reception staff, cleaning staff, recreation attendants and others hold a responsibility in other areas of the leisure facility, fitness staff hold responsibility for safety when the disabled person moves into, around and out of the space used for the fitness activity, and for ensuring appropriate supervision throughout the time spent within the fitness facility when exercising, as well as when not exercising.

It is necessary to anticipate the high level of care required when working with disabled people within a gym, exercise studio or any setting used for health and fitness activities. This is especially pertinent to smaller facilities that choose not to staff the gym at all times, or have only one member of staff on duty at any given time, requiring this individual to carry out pre-exercise screening, inductions, cleaning *and* monitoring of the facility while being sociable all at the same time! The fitness industry can require the ability to multi-task at a superhuman level! Adequate staffing is essential if accidents are to be avoided.

There are countless examples set out in law to show that the standard of care required need not necessarily be set out within the common practice regulations provided by the workplace. Appropriate inquiry and precaution must be taken, even if it is not common practice. Duty of care therefore also includes asking as many questions as necessary to gather information about the type and level of care required.

According to law, an employee cannot excuse a failure to meet the appropriate standard of care as a result of a lack of guidelines from within their facility. While policies and procedures should encompass the need for adaptation, they are often fairly rigid and set out in such a way that they assume all fitness facility users to be healthy. In fact, facility users are rarely completely free from aches, pains and medical conditions, and so adaptation is almost always required. We are all individuals and no two people are alike.

Duty of care lies not only in one direction, from the fitness instructor to the disabled person. It also holds for one participant to another, regardless of whether they have an impairment or not. A disabled person would be guilty of contributory negligence if they could have foreseen that a particular action – even if not directly involving them – might hurt or harm another person. That other person can be anyone with whom they come into contact, including the fitness instructors, other users and carers. If the fitness instructor believes that by allowing the disabled person to participate in the activity it would put others at risk, then under both the Health and Safety at Work Act and the DDA, they have the right to refuse participation. For example, it would be appropriate to refuse access to someone with a learning disability who was unable to provide a suitable care assistant, and who continued to hug fitness room users after having been asked to stop. Hugging someone who is holding a heavy weight could prove dangerous to all parties.

As with non-disabled people, a disabled person has a duty of care to himself or herself. A person is guilty of contributory negligence if they could have foreseen that a particular action might hurt them. For example, if the person senses that walking on a treadmill increases their knee pain, they have a duty to inform the instructor and ask whether this pain is appropriate. Similarly, if an instructor informs the participant that the leg extension machine is unsafe for them to use, they have a duty to follow the advice, asking for further explanation if required. Anyone participating in physical activity has a responsibility to follow instructions given and ask questions where there is a perceived danger.

If the disabled person does not have the ability to take this level of responsibility, they should be supervised throughout their session by someone who does. That supervisor must have an understanding of their client's needs, as they must take on the responsibility of making decisions and/or asking questions of the instructor on behalf of their client. It is essential that the supervisor fully understands the importance of their role if it requires them to take responsibility for the health and safety of the client. A parent, guardian or legal advocate will be aware of their legal responsibility, while a friend may not.

As the person with the greatest technical competence within the fitness environment, the fitness instructor has a duty to guide the supervisor and to exclude use of any equipment they deem unsuitable. While opposing opinions should always be heard, they should not be followed if they are deemed to be unsafe.

In some cases the instructor may realise that they are not qualified to carry out some of the requirements of the work with the particular participant, but they know of others who are. For example, the participant may wish to be carried from their wheelchair on to a workout bench. Without a lifting and handling qualification, the instructor should not take on this work. To do so would be to put themselves and the disabled participant at risk of serious injury and would certainly not be covered by insurance. Another example is where the participant requests assistance with personal care (going to the toilet, showering and/or changing). The instructor should refuse to carry out work for which they are unqualified, but they may be able to seek the assistance of another, such as a qualified carer. Simply requesting the presence of a carer can sometimes overcome these obstacles relatively easily. I work on the principle that nobody may have realised the need for assistance; and if you don't ask, you don't get!

In other cases the instructor may not be qualified to carry out any work at all with the particular participant. It may be possible to refer the client to another instructor who has the appropriate qualification. If there is no one appropriately qualified within your facility, it is useful to create contacts in other local facilities (possibly within the same company), creating a working relationship with such individuals to aid the referral process. Where no qualified instructor is available, refer the client to a medically trained person for further guidance.

Pre-Activity Readiness Questionnaire (PAR-Q)

All fitness instructors should be familiar with PAR-Qs. They come in many different shapes and sizes, designed and redesigned by in-house sales and marketing and/or programme managers. The recommended industry standard PAR-Q is based on one developed by the British Columbia Ministry of Health (revised by the Canadian Society for Exercise Physiology, 2002).

It is essential that a PAR-Q is completed by anyone and everyone before they commence physical activity. It is also essential that the information provided is read and analysed by someone appropriately trained. With facilities often being sales-driven, it may be those responsible for sales who are overseeing the completion of the PAR-Q. If they have not received training in the analysis of the form, then there is an immediate lapse in Duty of Care. Most importantly, it could put the disabled person at risk of illness or injury. Training should cover communication skills, to ensure there is sensitivity when asking personal questions, and pathways for referral if there are health concerns.

Forms that have only 'no' answers all the way through are known as negative, meaning there are no known health concerns that may cause a change in well being during or after exercise.

Any form that has 'yes' answers is known as a positive PAR-Q. It requires further investigation to find out if the client has misunderstood or misinterpreted any of the questions, or whether there may be health concerns. Further investigation needs to be managed sensitively and knowledgably, to build a sense of caring and confidence. The interviewer, having asked appropriate questions, then needs to ask themselves whether even further investigation is required.

If there is a need to gain greater insight, further probing is required with use of specific, closed questions. Questions may include:

- What medications are you taking?
- Do you have a named condition that causes your joint pain and, if so, what is its name?

If the questions cannot be understood or interpreted appropriately by the disabled person, an interpreter, carer or advocate should be used to assist. Questions should be asked directly to the disabled person and their responses noted before listening to the responses of the assistant.

If questioning confirms that the PAR-Q is positive, referral to a medically trained professional is required. The manner in which this is handled can make all the difference to the client. While many will perceive that referral creates barriers to exercise, it is important to explain how the system is designed to offer care and prevent medical emergencies or the worsening of current conditions.

Case Study

In spring 2006, a man who had been referred by his GP to a council gym to assist with a weight-loss plan was referred back because his blood-pressure reading was high. He was annoyed by this, believing the facility to be 'fat-ist' in their approach. It would seem that some of the national press, who reported this story, agreed with him. For example, in the *Metro* newspaper the headline to the article was, 'You're far too fat to work out in our gym'.

The man did not join the council gym, but without further investigation was accepted for membership by a private health club. Should the man have had a medical emergency while on their premises, the private club would have been liable for negligence, having not followed up on a known risk factor.

Work closely with those involved in referral schemes to create links with helpful GPs, practice nurses and physiotherapists. Ensure you give useful, friendly advice. It is worthwhile having ready-prepared letters for referral, both for the client and for the medical practitioner. The letter to the medical practitioner should be sent on headed paper, with full contact details, an explanation of why the letter is being sent and exactly what information is required.

Ensure that permission to exercise by a medically qualified person is given in writing. Read the return letter carefully, ensuring you receive an original copy so that you are able to check the authenticity. If the referee has made recommendations, these must be followed.

Some referees will not give permission to exercise. In this case, the client must be refused access. This seems harsh, but it is to protect both the client and the instructor. Think what it would feel like if there were a medical emergency resulting from non-compliance with these recommendations. Try to offer other exercise solutions, through links with specialist services such as cardiac rehabilitation and falls-prevention. The more information you have available about local specialist services, the better prepared you will feel and the more helpful you can be.

Finally, note that the standard PAR-Q may not give all the health information you need when programming exercise. People with medical conditions may have a negative PAR-Q. Therefore, be prepared to ask further questions. The more information you have about your clients, the more tailored to their individual needs the programme can be.

Pre-activity assessment

Pre-activity assessment, otherwise known as fitness assessment, is a helpful tool to find out more about your client than can be gained from initial questioning.

If the pre-activity assessment is to be effective, it must have relevance to the client and to the instructor. It should provide personalised information on the following areas:

- The impairment(s) and the effect of this on the individual
- The medication(s) and the effect of this on the individual
- Why the client wants to exercise – their goals
- How the client would prefer to exercise, for example in an exercise class, gym, at home, or outdoors
- Exercise history
- Current lifestyle – activity levels and time availability
- Support required for success of the exercise programme
- Current level of function.

With practice, it should be possible to gather all of the above information within 30 minutes. At first it may take longer, but as knowledge and skill develop, so does effective use of time.

It may be that, having completed the assessment, further technical questions about the client's impairments are raised. As previously stated, referral to a medically trained individual may be required. Alternatively, it may be that time needs to be taken to carry out research before further client contact.

Many disabled people attending health and fitness sessions for the first time will have a very low level of fitness. Full information needs to be gathered to help understand what reduced function there may be and whether this reduced function is due to a lack of fitness or due to the impairment. The instructor should consider whether a fitness programme is capable of improving function or whether the loss is permanent and is incapable of being improved by physical activity.

Information about the impairment and medication may be indicated on the PAR-Q. This depends on the type of questions on the PAR-Q used within your facility. Further questioning is likely to be required, regardless of this. While open questions can provide a good start, closed questions may be needed to gain the exact information required.

Open questions may include:

- How does your impairment affect you?
- What can you tell me about your medical condition?

Closed questions may then be required to gain further insight specific to the needs of the instructor. Examples are:

- Can you stand up independently?
- Can you move your legs at all? Please show me.
- Can you hold a pen?

A discussion about the goals of a new exercise programme is important at this stage (*see* the section on goal setting, pages 38–43).

Once as much information as possible has been gained from questioning, it is helpful to commence a functional assessment. This will give much more information about the individual, including:

- The starting fitness level of the individual
- The starting ability level of the individual related to each of their goals

- How any impairment is likely to affect their ability to participate
- The exact amount of movement at those joints affected by the impairment
- The ability to comprehend instructions
- The ability to interpret and carry out instructions
- The type of equipment, if any, that is most appropriate
- The type of equipment that is inappropriate.

Traditionally, the health and fitness industry has taken standardised measures at initial assessment, including blood pressure, height, weight, body fat percentage, peak flow (an indication of lung function) and sub-maximal VO_2 (an indication of cardiovascular fitness). While results from these measures may have some meaning to the instructor, they rarely have meaning for the client, other than to confirm their unfitness!

For some disabled clients, norm tables will have no relevance. Prediction of body mass, lung function and VO_2 max are all affected by amputated limbs, lack of limb development, muscle wastage and neurological deficits affecting muscular performance. Additionally, if a client has a condition affecting their comprehension or motivation (such as a stroke or learning disabilities), their test performance will be affected and a falsely low result will be obtained.

In recent years, arm ergometer tests have been developed for use with clients who cannot complete tests of cardiovascular performance using their legs. While these can be useful within laboratory sports science testing, their relevance is limited within gyms, as the muscular activity often does not have relevance to activities of daily living (ADLs) and norm tables can be misleading.

Each measure should be explained in language that can be easily understood by the client. It should relate to them personally, rather than to a textbook. I cannot remember a single client who has ever become excited by knowing their sub-maximal VO_2 max score. By contrast, many clients have become motivated by learning about their ability to perform life-related tasks and knowing that, by measuring these at regular intervals (usually every six to eight weeks), we can both be sure about whether the exercise programme is having a positive impact upon their lives.

Use of language within assessment tools is equally important. For example, while the word 'flexibility' is commonly used within the industry, this can have more meaning if reframed as, for example, the ability to reach to a high shelf or do up your shoes. While I might be performing what I would term a flexibility test, I can reframe it to the client as a test to measure the ability to do something tangible and relevant.

Funding agencies are becoming increasingly keen to receive feedback on the performance of the projects they fund. In the past, anecdotal qualitative feedback has often been sufficient. Summaries of comments and ratings scores on feedback forms have been the most common way of showing success. However, following guidance from NICE, there is now a preference for more objective, quantitative feedback in addition to the qualitative. This means that exact measurements are required to show the deemed success or failure of the project. Examples of measures that provide quantitative feedback are:

- body fat percentage: the percentage of body fat reduction in those attending due to obesity
- timed walk: the number of participants who are able to improve by ten seconds the time they take to walk five metres.

Throughout the process of assessment, motivational interviewing techniques should be utilised (*see* page 43).

Only once there has been a full assessment process is it possible to gain a fair understanding of each client's physical, psychological and sociological make-up. By taking the time to gain this information at the outset, time will be used more effectively from then onwards, as it will be possible to prepare a truly individualised programme.

Example assessment measures

Blood pressure

A blood pressure reading is the only assessment measure always recommended before exercising commences, since high blood pressure (hypertension) often has no sign or symptom and most exercise is likely to slightly raise blood pressure. All other assessment measures should be selected according to the individual.

Posture

Another extremely useful measure is standing or seated posture. Carefully observe the client in a static standing or seated position and make a note of any asymmetry between left and right sides and whether there are any obvious changes to ideal posture (*see* pages 110–1). Report your findings back to the client and see if together you can find any obvious reasons for imbalances.

Functional measures

Table 3.1 gives examples of some functional assessment measures. This is by no means a complete list. Talking to your clients about their goals will give you ideas about what to measure, so that the assessment process becomes useful and meaningful to each individual.

> **Top tips for fitness assessment**
>
> Consider the purpose behind each measure and check that it has relevance to:
> - the individual;
> - exercise selection;
> - setting the intensity of each exercise;
> - monitoring the achievement of goals.
>
> Ensure that the results from each measure are explained to the client using jargon-free language.

The environment

The suitability of the environment to be used by disabled participants must be taken into consideration. Legally, a suitable area must be made available. This may require the assistance of other participants, especially in areas where loose equipment is left around. Health and safety law not only provides for the requirements of instructors, but also for anyone who may come into contact with other users.

Table 3.1	Sample functional assessments
1 Timed up and go (measure of standing balance and walking function)	Ask the client to sit on a firm, upright chair. Time the client from the moment they start to stand up, as they walk 5m to a distance marker, as they return back to the chair, and stop the clock once they have sat down. Repeat. Record both times; make notes about walking aids and technique.
2 Sit to stand (measure of quadriceps power and ability to get up from a chair)	Record the number of times the client can sit to stand in one minute. Take notes about technique.
3 Shoulder flexibility (measure of shoulder range of movement for life-related tasks)	Measure the height the client can reach to up a wall; measure how far their hand will reach over their shoulder and down their back. Measure both sides.
4 Six-minute walk (measure of cardiovascular endurance)	Measure the distance covered when walking around a set course for six minutes, either measuring the distance or the number of laps. Make notes about walking aids and technique.
6 Pain/energy scale (measure of 'coping' ability)	Ask the client to mark a cross on the 10cm line below to show how much pain interferes with everyday life and/or how much energy they have in the morning/evening.

Top tips for creating suitable fitness environments

Within fitness studios, attention should be paid to the following:

- Level of flooring: monitor travel across uneven surfaces
- Wet flooring: monitor floors that become slippery when wet (from sweat and/or spilt drinks) and dry them or clear them accordingly
- Spare equipment: store away from the exercising area when not in use
- Used equipment: lay out in a manner that does not interfere with safe movement to, from and within the workout area
- Arrangement of class participants: organise participants to stand or sit in a particular arrangement if this may influence their health and safety
- Volume of music: ensure the instructor's voice can be heard above the music.

Within gyms, attention should be paid to the above, plus in addition:

- Arrangement of fixed machinery: consider layout so that there are no trip hazards and there is sufficient space to manoeuvre a wheelchair.

If wheelchair users are to be able to use an area, there should be space for manoeuvring the wheelchair. Space should also be available for parking the wheelchair while the person transfers to each machine to exercise. Some wheelchair users will be able to walk, so space should be provided beside at least one treadmill and one bike, as well as resistance machines and rowing machines.

PRINCIPLES OF FITNESS PROGRAMMING

Programming tools

Experienced instructors will find their own methods to ensure that the programmes they prepare for their clients are tailored to the individual's requirements and goals. Various programming tools can be used to assist with this. They enable a methodical, consistent approach and also provide a system by which the instructor can check that all necessary information is provided.

In order to ensure that all avenues have been covered, it can be helpful to follow a set structure when writing a programme. Whether or not you use the framework suggested below to start writing your programmes or to make checks once you have finished, it is important to follow a process that works for you.

A complete programme is one that addresses information covering the following areas:

- F   frequency
- I   intensity
- T   time
- T   type
- A   adherence

Frequency: how often the whole programme and each exercise within the programme should be completed, usually per week.
Intensity: how hard each exercise and the overall programme should feel.
Time: how long each exercise and the overall programme should take.
Type: what exercises should be completed and in what order.
Adherence: whether the programme addresses individual goals and psychological needs as well as physical needs.

It is essential to keep the goals of each client in mind as you prepare the programme, as your client tries it out and as the client continues to use it. It can be helpful to write the goals at the top of any programme card, to act as a frequent reminder to you and your client. In this way not only do you both remain focussed, but in the very busy world of a fitness instructor you are provided with a quick reminder of the individual, their needs and wants.

The purpose of each and every exercise within the programme should be known. It is just not good enough to simply include bicep curls within every programme because you find them easy to instruct! An ability to express verbally the purpose in both a technical and a non-technical manner will aid communication with colleagues and with the client. Consideration of who is being communicated with and what is trying to be communicated can be helpful. For example, the purpose of a shoulder press may be expressed in the following two ways:

- To improve the strength of the triceps and anterior deltoid (technical).
- To improve the ability to reach for objects on high shelves (non-technical).

The purpose of an exercise may be:

- Physical: for example, to improve the ability to stand up from a chair independently
- Psychological: for example, to calm down over-excitement
- A mix of both: for example, to improve gait (walking ability) while also maintaining concentration/improving confidence.

The final programme should be useable by a colleague without them having to ask for your interpretation. It should therefore use industry-standard language. Also consider whether you are trying to promote client independence. If so, attention should be paid to ensuring the programme is delivered in a user-friendly manner, with industry jargon de-jargonised. After working in the industry for only a short period of time, most instructors become so used to industry jargon that they no longer recognise it as jargon. For example, consider how many of your facility users understand the terms 'developmental stretch' or 'overload', or know the names of the muscles they are working. It may be that you are able to explain these terms verbally and/or in writing, or it may be that words can be replaced with pictures or symbols.

While client-centred programming can at first appear time-consuming, it makes the job of a fitness instructor extremely interesting. No two programmes should ever appear the same again. Variety relieves boredom and is the spice of life!

Intensity-monitoring

It is important to make a decision about how intense the workout should feel for the client at any given time. In this way it is possible to not only ask the client how intense it feels, but also know whether their response is more than ideal, less than ideal or just perfect!

For many people who are new to exercise, the feeling of an increased heart rate can be quite scary. This is especially so for people who are nervous of the fitness environment, who may even perceive the feeling of their heart beating faster to be the onset of a panic attack. Clearly this would be extremely frightening.

Consideration of intensity-monitoring at the programming stage will enable effective measurement and setting of intensities at the first session. Exercise intensity can be monitored either by use of pulse-rate monitoring or a rate of perceived exertion (RPE) scale.

Pulse-rate monitoring is often the most precise tool for monitoring. However, there are situations in which it should not be used, or only used with caution:

- Certain medications limit heart rate levels so that the pulse rate will not increase proportionally with exercise intensity;
- Conventional formulae for working out MHR and percentage of this are inappropriate and provide incorrect information for individuals with loss of muscular function;
- Some people will find the use of a chest strap invasive, frightening or uncomfortable;
- Some individuals will be unable to understand the information.

While there are several validated RPE scales commonly used within the fitness industry, when working with disabled people these may not always work. The validated Borg and adapted Borg scales use a numbering system. If working with a client who finds it difficult to understand or interpret a scale communicated using numbers, consider using alternative units. Smiling to frowning faces, thumb-up through to thumb-down positions, colour shades or even likes and dislikes (as shown in Table 3.2) can provide an easy-to-comprehend alternative. Although not scientifically validated, if they are understood by the client then they do the job. Not only do they enable intensity feedback to be communicated between the instructor and the client, but they allow intensity to be interpreted in a manner that encourages independence. This is all about thinking in a client-centred manner.

Intensity can be adjusted in a number of ways using the Five Rs:

- Repetition
- Resistance

Table 3.2	Examples of RPE scales						
Very Very light	Very light	Fairly light	Some-what hard	Hard	Very hard	Very very hard
6 7	8 9	10 11 12	13 14	15 16	17 18	19 20
Easy			Average			Hard
1	2 3	4 5	6	7	8 9	10
☺			☻			☹
🖐			☞			🖐
Pink		Purple		Blue		Green
Chocolate		*EastEnders*		Swimming		Beef stew

- Range of movement
- Rest
- Rate

Repetitions: the number of times an exercise is performed, either with or without a rest in between.

Resistance: the amount of exertion required to move the body or an object.

Range of movement: the range one or more joints goes through to complete each movement.

Rest (or recovery): the time in which intensity is lowered (active rest) or stopped (between each exercise during the exercise session and between each exercise session).

Rate (or speed): the speed at which each exercise is performed.

Although changing the type of exercise also changes the intensity, it is actually the change in one or more of the 'Rs' inherent within each exercise that creates the intensity difference.

Figure 3.2 shows how changes in any 'R' affects exercise intensity and therefore how to progress an exercise. The arrows indicate change in level of intensity. For example, if repetitions are increased, both CV and resistance exercises become more intense. Note that if rate is increased, CV exercise becomes harder but resistance exercise becomes easier. Unlike all the others, these arrows point in opposing directions.

Figure 3.2 The five 'Rs' of exercise Intensity

If each of the Rs is increased:

	CV	Resistance
Repetitions	↑	↑
Resistance	↑	↑
Range of movement	↑	↑
Rest	↓	↓
Rate	↑	↓

Of the Five Rs, repetitions and resistance are the most commonly used by gym instructors to adjust intensity, perhaps mainly because programme cards make it easy to note the levels of these. Within the studio environment, exercise to music instructors are particularly good at adjusting range of movement, using the beats of the music to inspire larger (as well as faster) movements, while circuit training instructors are well known for their ability to work with rest by using a timed work-to-rest ratio. Fitness instructors who teach all of these types of sessions are well placed to offer the best of each. Every exercise programme should contain information about all five Rs.

Which to alter first is, as always, dependent on the individual client's needs. If a disabled client finds it difficult to lift their arm or move their leg through sufficient range to cope with life-related movement, this should almost always be the first of the Rs to be worked upon. There is no point in being able to lift an increasingly heavy weight through a tiny range of movement, but improving the range so that the individual increases their independence is life changing.

To make any exercise easier or harder, it is likely that no more than one or two Rs should be altered.

Components of an exercise programme

A usual health-related exercise programme should include the following components:

- Warm-up
- Cardiovascular training
- Resistance training
- Cool down.

These should address the five components of fitness, these being (in no particular order):

- Cardiovascular fitness
- Muscular strength
- Muscular endurance
- Flexibility
- Motor skills/co-ordination.

When working with disabled people, there may be limitations on duration and intensity of exercise that require the usual programme to be adapted. This will be as a direct result of the medical conditions and/or the medications the individual is taking. In principle, duration and intensity are limited by the energy expenditure involved in an activity. Mechanical efficiency, or the ability to perform a movement utilising the minimum amount of energy, is impaired and increased by the following factors:

Pain

Consider how tired and grumpy you become when you have been in pain! Now consider how much earlier fatigue will set in for people who attempt to exercise through the pain.

Obesity

Excess fat must be carried along with lean tissue as the individual moves. To the person's body, it is as if they were permanently holding a set of weights.

Nerve dysfunction and muscle paralysis

Damage to nerves interrupts the flow of information from the brain to the muscle. Where one or more muscles across a joint are paralysed, those that still function will have to work even harder to bring about movement. In some cases, messages may have the opportunity to get through, but may take longer or may be weaker. In such instances, more concentration is required to bring about a required movement.

Nerve dysfunction and muscle spasticity

Where one or more muscles across a joint constantly have tension through them, metabolic activity is increased and greater effort is required to move through required planes of movement.

Poor posture

If there is an unstable base, greater effort is required to bring about controlled limb movement.

Low body awareness and proprioception

Anyone who has difficulty in balance, or in knowing how to go about moving one or more limbs through certain planes, will need to put in more physical effort and greater concentration levels.

Depression

Low mood can cause loss of concentration and focus.

Fear or anxiety

These can result due to a decreased ability to perform an activity, especially if this increases the risk of falling or colliding, or due to discomfort with the surroundings. Being in a state of fear or anxiety sets off primal systems in our bodies that are there to protect us whenever we feel threatened or in danger. Hormones are released that are designed to excite. As a result, concentration levels are usually heightened to make the mind alert (ready for fight) and the heart rate increases (ready for flight). Even at low intensities, the body will be working hard and therefore it will run out of steam even after only small amounts of effort. Could this be why so many people new to your fitness session tire quickly, but comment on their improvement within two to three sessions?

Consider how it must feel for a disabled person, new to exercise and scared that they 'don't fit in', who is overweight and has a condition that causes pain or muscle dysfunction. Is it any wonder that they fatigue quickly? An appreciation of their physical and psychological abilities must be reflected within the programme. We should be in awe of anyone who fits into this category, who turns up repeatedly and learns to enjoy the fitness environment into the long term.

Duration and intensity limitations may mean that one or more programme and/or fitness components need to be omitted. Careful consideration needs to be taken to ensure that the final programme is safe as well as effective. For example, for safety reasons the warm-up is usually an essential programme component, while the resistance component could be omitted.

Warm-up

The content and duration of a warm-up will vary according to the fitness level and health of each individual. In principle, a warm-up should consist of a mobility component, a pulse raiser component and a stretch component. However, the amount of time spent on each of these and even whether they are actually included at all is completely individual.

Mobility and Pulse-Raiser

For those who have a very low level of fitness, the warm-up needs to be very long – up to 20 minutes in duration. There are various reasons for this:

- **The circulatory system**: Individuals who have cardiovascular diseases or are sedentary, spending long periods sitting still, often have a very poorly functioning circulatory system. When exercise is commenced, even at a very low intensity, a high amount of stress is put on the circulatory system as it attempts to redistribute blood to the working muscles. Movement should be continued for as long as it takes to redistribute blood safely and effectively, to warm and energise the muscles to be used in the main workout.

- **Joint mobility**: People with joint conditions may require additional time spent on mobilising the joint or joints affected. Sedentary individuals also tend to stiffen up, so much so that they will frequently complain of joint pain and may be slow and unstable in their movements. Great care must be taken to gradually introduce movement within a pain-free range. Small movements may need to be repeated before synovial fluid can start to lubricate the joint sufficiently to introduce larger movements. Non-weight-bearing exercises, otherwise known as seated exercises, can help to reduce the need to concentrate on balance and can reduce the risk of increasing pain levels at the onset of exercise.

- **Body awareness**: Those with little or no past experience of exercise, and those with a neurological or cognitive condition, can find it difficult to appreciate what it feels like to move their body through certain planes or patterns of movement and through the full range that is available. A slow rehearsal of these planes or patterns, which could include basic movements required in everyday life, can be helpful to educate, inform and prepare for the main workout.

The difficulty in achieving a sufficient duration of warm-up is that after two to three minutes the participant may complain of exhaustion, even when exercising at the lowest of intensities. It is unsafe to simply end the warm-up early and go straight into the main workout, as neither the mind nor the body will be sufficiently prepared. In such cases, the skill is to offer active rests by mixing the pulse raiser and mobility together. The term 'active rests' is used to convey the principle of maintaining movement, but at a level of intensity that is relatively easy for the participant.

The ideal warm-up for someone with a very low level of fitness is to start with small-range, seated pulse raising, such as can be achieved through chair-based exercise or a recumbent bike. After two to three minutes, introduce 6-10 repetitions of a mobility exercise. Ensure there are sufficient repetitions of the selected exercise to effectively mobilise, but not so many as to fatigue the muscles crossing the joints involved. Restart the pulse raising and continue to stop at two- to three-minute intervals to complete different mobility exercises. Repeat a sequence as many times and for as long as is required.

Sample mobility and pulse raiser warm-ups can be seen in figure 3.3.

Sample 1: Seated, for someone with no function of leg or lumbar spine muscles.

1 Posture – using back support
2 Bicep curls x 10
3 Arm swings x 10
4 Shoulder rolls x 10
5 Low 'slap and clap' x 10
6 Neck turns x 10
7 Marching x 10
8 High 'slap and clap' x 10
9 Repeat the above with greater range of movement and/or speed.

Figure 3.3 Sample mobility and pulse-raisers

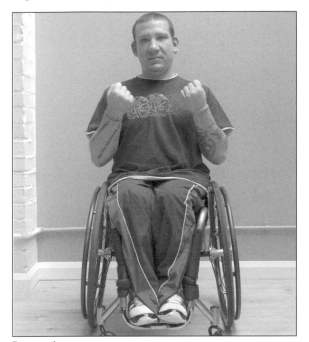
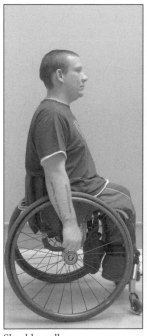

Bicep curls

Shoulder rolls

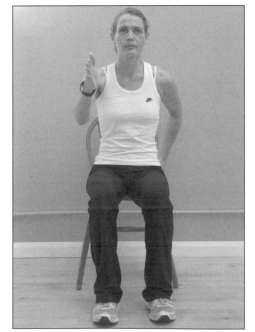
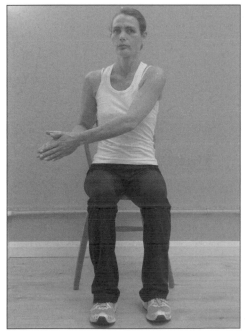

Arm swings

Low slap and clap

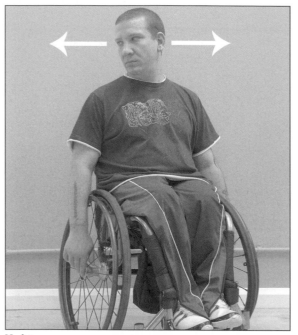

Neck turns

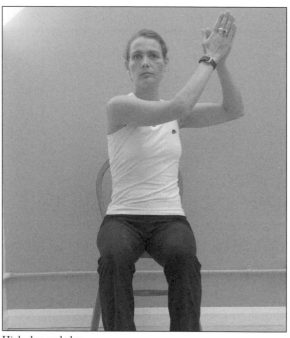

High slap and clap

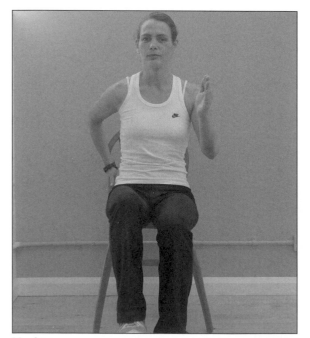

Marching

Sample 2: Seated, for someone unable to stand up, but with leg function (include posture breaks, sitting to the back of the chair, as required).

1 Posture – sitting to the front third of the chair
2 Heel lifts x 30 sec
3 Arm swings x 30 sec
4 Repeat 2 and 3
5 Marching x 30 sec
6 Shoulder rolls x 8
7 Marching x 30 sec
8 Side bends x 8
9 Marching x 30 sec
10 Trunk twists x 8
11 Marching x 30 sec
12 Ankle point and flex x 8

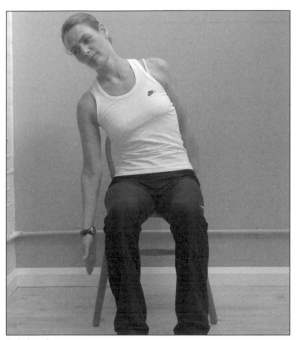

Side bends

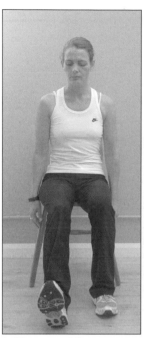

Ankle point and flex

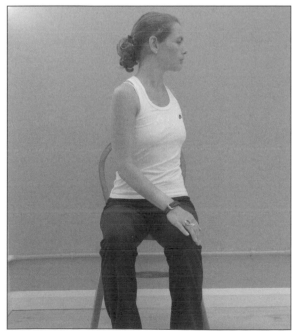

Trunk twists

Sample 3: Seated using CV equipment, for someone with poor leg mobility.

1 Posture
2 Recumbent bike (bent knees, ignore screen set-up) x 2 min
3 Move feet out of pedals on to floor; seated arm swings x 30 sec
4 Recumbent bike (bent knees, ignore screen set-up) x 2 min
5 Move feet on to floor; seated shoulder rolls x 8
6 Recumbent bike (move seat back one hole, ignore screen set-up) x 2 min
7 Move feet out of pedals on to floor; seated side bends x 8
8 Recumbent bike x 2 min
9 Move feet to floor; seated trunk twists x 8
10 Recumbent bike x 2 min

If this takes up to 20 minutes to be effective, it may be enough of a workout on its own. Certainly there will be no requirement for a separate cardiovascular component. Then, as the participant gains in fitness, time saved during the warm-up can be spent on a longer main component, possibly with the introduction of a cardiovascular component.

A fitter individual, although able to work at a higher intensity in the main workout, will be able to use the improved cardiovascular ability to pulse-raise more quickly. Therefore, although a higher intensity is required to achieve a warming effect, it should take less time to get safely to that level of intensity.

Pre-Stretch

Stretching before a main workout has received bad press over recent years. However, it is important to consider the needs of each individual client. If the individual has correct muscle balance/posture and good body awareness, stretching would not be necessary and would be an ineffective use of time.

The majority of disabled people will have one or more of the following that makes a pre-stretch of one or more muscles an important component of the warm-up:

• **Poor body awareness**, so that full range of movement is not utilised. It is almost as if the individual has forgotten the reach to which their body is capable. Practising through the full range, either with static stretches (held at the end of the range) or dynamic stretches (slow, controlled movement repeated up to five times through the range) may re-educate or remind the person of their capabilities.

• **Muscle imbalance**, so that partner muscles pull the body out of correct alignment. Most muscles work in groups, with action brought about by a prime mover and synergists (or partners). Sometimes synergists become too active, taking over from what should be the prime mover. Stretching muscles that are too strong will reduce their working capability, forcing the relatively weak muscles in the group to carry out a proportionally greater amount of the work.

• **Poor flexibility** generally throughout the body. If increased flexibility is one of the main goals of exercising, use regular opportunities within the workout to improve it and to familiarise the participant with stretches that can be practised regularly at home.

Dependent on the individual requirements, if a pre-stretch is to be included, consider which muscles to stretch, for how long and in what position. Some considerations are explained in table 3.3 on page 77.

Table 3.3	Stretch considerations

1 If the goal of the stretch is to challenge balance while taking the joint to the end of its range, it may be appropriate to keep the individual in a standing position.

2 If the goal is solely to take the joint to the end of its range, a seated or lying option may be more appropriate.

3 If the goal of stretching a muscle is to 'switch it off' to encourage other lazy muscles to work harder, a static stretch duration of at least 20 seconds is required.

4 If the goal is to improve body awareness, a static stretch duration of 10 seconds is sufficient.

5 Usually, one repetition of each static stretch or five repetitions of a dynamic stretch is sufficient in the warm-up.

6 Lying options are often inappropriate early in the workout as they encourage relaxation of mood as well as of body.

Examples of dynamic stretches suitable in the warm-up not only for stretching but also for improving co-ordination (improved movement pathways) can be seen in Figure 3.4 on pages 78–80.

Examples of standing, seated and lying static stretch positions can be seen in figure 3.6 on page 85.

Case study

A profoundly deaf six-foot male, aged 25, has a kyphotic posture but is otherwise healthy. Would you include a pre-stretch in his programme and, if so, would you stretch muscles to the front and muscles to the back of the upper torso? I would suggest that to help realign his posture he should perform a developmental stretch for his chest muscles, anterior deltoid and any other muscles (such as his hamstrings) that might be indicated in his poor posture. I would not stretch any other muscles.

Main workout – Cardiovascular and resistance training

Within the main workout, consider again the function of each exercise related to the individual you are training. In everyday life different types of muscular activity are required, including:

- Explosive power – the ability to perform once with the greatest effort and speed;
- Anaerobic power – the ability to perform a few times with high effort;
- Anerobic capacity – the ability to perform for up to two minutes;
- Aerobic capacity – the ability to perform over an extended period.

Each of these should be taken into consideration when preparing a programme. In addition, consider whether motor skills/co-ordination is a component of fitness that requires training. If so, this must be addressed within the cardiovascular (CV) and/or resistance sections.

Ensure attention is paid to appropriate exercise specificity. For example, if the goal is to improve the client's walking skills, there must be some walking involved; a bike will

Figure 3.4 Dynamic warm-up stretches

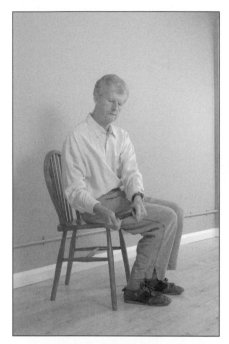
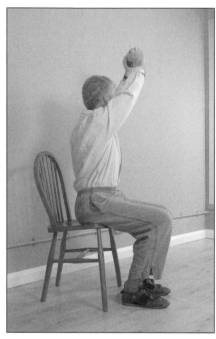
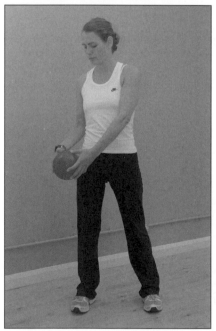
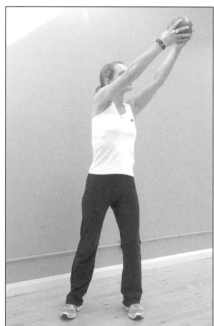

Seated/standing unweighted ball diagonal plane

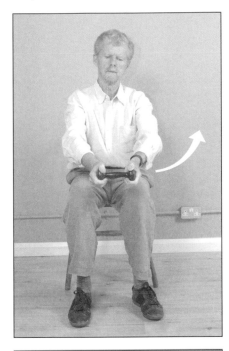
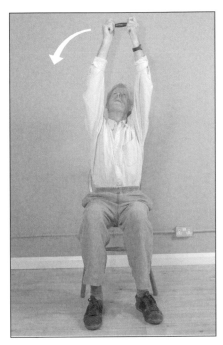

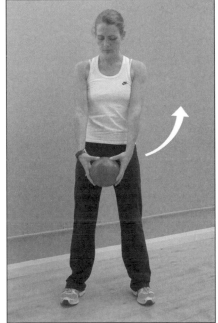
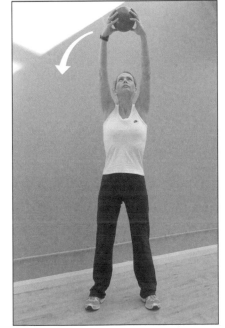

Seated/standing unweighted ball circles

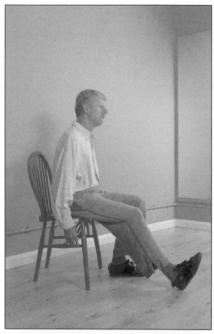
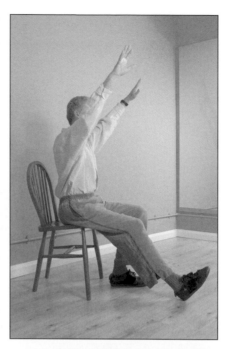
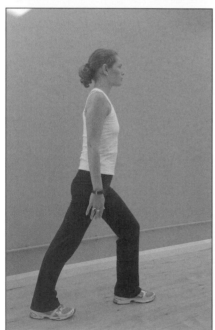
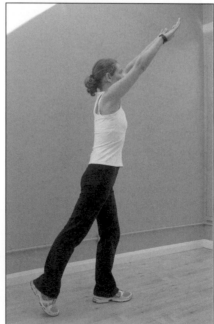

Seated/standing dynamic calf/arm stretch

not improve walking skills. Or if the goal is to improve their standing balance, there should be some standing; again using a bike will not improve the ability to stand. Although this may sound fairly obvious, the client's expectations about use of equipment may inappropriately cause a loss of focus on identified goals.

Link the information given within this chapter with information about the medical conditions (*see* Chapter 19) and how they affect your client. For example, people with some medical conditions should never exercise to either overall fatigue or fatigue on specific individual exercises. These guidelines provide a basis for further questioning and should not be used on their own. Remember, if you overview the programme you prepare using the FITTA principles, you will be sure to encompass individual needs and wants.

While it is usually fairly obvious whether an exercise is for CV or resistance training, it can be less obvious when working with individuals who have limited function. Consider whether the exercise is fatiguing the individual's CV system by gaining feedback on their breathing rate and/or pulse rate. Consider whether the exercise is fatiguing the individual's muscular system by gaining feedback on the energy left in the muscle.

By gaining this feedback, it is possible to find out which system limits the continuation of the exercise – the CV system or the muscular system. An exercise that is for CV benefit for one person may well be for muscular benefit for another. For example, squats are conventionally given as resistance training but, if the exerciser becomes breathless before muscle fatigue sets in, they may well be re-classified as a CV exercise. Sidesteps are conventionally given as a CV exercise but, if the exerciser mentions

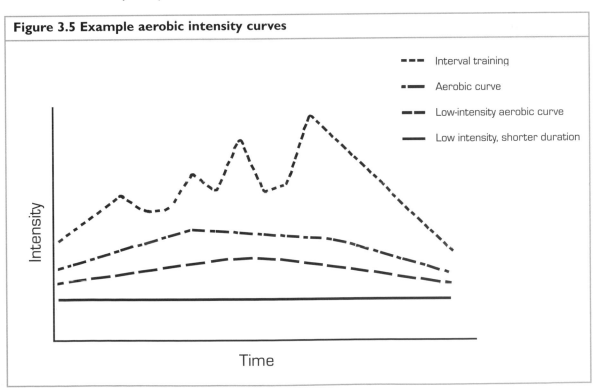

Figure 3.5 Example aerobic intensity curves

- - - Interval training

■-■ Aerobic curve

■ ■ Low-intensity aerobic curve

—— Low intensity, shorter duration

Intensity

Time

fatigue of leg muscles without any obvious change in breathing rate, they may be re-classified as a resistance exercise.

There are no set rules about whether the CV section should be performed before or after the resistance section. A decision should be made based on the individual's goals, health and fitness levels. Indeed, it may be more appropriate to mix up these two components of the session, using resistance exercises as active rest periods between the CV exercises. This can be effective not only for those with low cardiovascular fitness, but also for those who have a short concentration span.

Cardiovascular

Although there are a few basic principles to be followed, the specific nature of this section will vary. Informed decisions must be made about duration, intensity and the type of activities to be performed. Think FITTA principles.

There should always be a pulse-raiser to build intensity, and the pulse should always be lowered at the end. Whether a section is required between these to maintain the pulse, and how much intensity builds, is dependent on the aerobic and/or anaerobic capacities of the individual. A client who has low cardiovascular fitness may show an aerobic straight, where the intensity is more or less maintained, rather than an aerobic curve, where intensity is raised, maintained and then lowered (*see* fig. 3.5).

As with all clients, ensure intensity is raised and lowered gradually. For de-conditioned individuals this may take longer than expected and could involve what may have previously been considered to be very low-intensity activity. *Oxygen debt*, the depletion of oxygen levels available within the body to a level where cells are in constant catch-up, will soon set in with de-conditioned individuals who maintain a constant low intensity.

Any exercise which increases the pulse rate, but can be maintained, and includes rhythmic, continuous movements involving use of large muscle groups, can be considered to be a CV exercise. Typical and less typical CV exercises can be seen in table 3.4.

It may be necessary to adapt your conventional thinking to accommodate different individuals, especially those with a loss of leg function. Where there is a loss of

Table 3.4	CV exercises
Typical	**Untypical**
Walking	Weight training exercises (light resistance, high repetitions e.g. x 50)
Running	Chest press
Swimming	Lat pulldown
Cycling	Leg press
Rowing	
Arm ergometer	
Aerobics	
Step	

function in one or both legs, there will be a loss of use of the largest muscle groups in the body. In order to maximise the potential demand for oxygen, consider where the next-largest working muscles are and try to use these. In the upper body, the trapezius, latissimus dorsi and pectoralis major are usually good choices.

Normal wheelchair-pushing may provide a limited training stimulus for the cardiovascular system, as various studies have found that pulse rate increases to no more than 55 per cent MHR. This is because wheelchair users must employ their arm muscles to exercise, and these by definition are smaller than leg muscles, requiring less oxygen to fuel their movement. A greater effort is required, either by increasing the speed of pushing or the force applied to each push, or by altering the terrain (gradient, type of surface).

When arm muscles are used there is a much smaller margin between training overload that causes improved fitness and training overload that causes injury. Various studies have looked at the oxygen cost of arm ergometry compared to leg ergometry and have found it to be substantially higher, by up to 33 per cent. This is believed to be due to the increased amount of effort required to stabilise the trunk, as there is a proportionally lowered increase in oxygen consumption in people with higher levels of spinal cord lesion who have lost the ability to control trunk stabiliser muscles.

Constant monitoring of intensity, either using pulse rate monitoring or an RPE scale (see pages 68–70) is essential. Talk testing and observation of client performance are good indicators but are not sufficiently accurate, nor do they assist the client to become independent and responsible for monitoring intensity by themselves. Talk testing and observation should always be used when working with a client, but in addition rather than instead of pulse rate monitoring or an RPE scale.

Resistance

For each exercise, there are a huge range of considerations, including:

- What needs to be trained – one or more muscles, one or more movements?
- Whether the goal of the exercise is muscular strength or muscular endurance;
- Whether an element of co-ordination is to be trained;
- Whether there is a life-related aim behind it;
- Whether training should or should not be to fatigue or even failure;
- Whether the same muscles should be worked with different exercises (supersets);
- Whether to perform one or more sets of the same exercise;
- In what order the exercises should be performed.

In order to make accurate decisions, especially about the level of resistance, communication with the client is essential. Although the instructor should have an idea about the type and order of exercises and the number of repetitions of each, final decisions about the level of resistance are unlikely to be known without utilising a system of trial and error as the client attempts each exercise. Once again, a system of intensity monitoring must be used. Use one of those previously suggested (see pages 68–70).

Cool-down

The content of a cool-down will vary depending on the content of the main workout. Suffice it to say, a cool-down is almost always essential, the only exception being when the exerciser becomes suddenly fatigued, suggesting that more activity of any kind would not be in their best interests and might be unsafe.

Case study

A 65-year-old male client, relatively new to exercise, with a condition that causes tremor when fatigue sets in, mentioned that he was finding it increasingly difficult to lift books on to the shelves when at work. He would attempt to 'throw' books on to shelves once they had been used, and his secretary would tidy up those that had missed at the end of each day!

Although it was clear that the client needed to do some strength-biased training, I had to be cautious about setting off the tremor. I set a resistance for each exercise that I thought the client might be able to lift no more than 12 times and after eight repetitions asked him how many more repetitions he thought he might be able to lift. I then asked him to stop at two repetitions fewer than he had said, therefore stopping before he thought he would reach failure.

If the pulse or workout intensity is relatively high for the individual at the end of the main workout, then a CV-biased exercise to gradually lower intensity is required. It may also be advisable if a smooth, rhythmical activity will assist in calming the mind of a participant who has become excited by the relatively high demands of the main workout. If the end of the main workout has involved relatively slow activity and the individual has cooled down, then a CV-biased exercise to increase circulation and re-warm is required. The decision as to whether to start the cool-down with a CV-biased exercise may vary from day to day, according to the individual's energy and pain levels. It is important to ensure that any decision made is well considered and to check it meets the individual's needs on that specific occasion.

Once the individual is sufficiently calmed and/or warm, consider a post-workout stretch to maintain and/or improve flexibility. This is the ideal time in the workout to work on flexibility, as no further demands are to be made on the body or the mind.

Consideration needs to be given to which muscles to stretch and for what purpose. Each individual will vary in their need, with some needing muscles stretched to aid rebalance or posture, and others not requiring any stretches at all. An individual with hypermobile joints should not stretch the muscles crossing those joints, as this would only encourage the joints to become even more unstable. Stretch those muscles that need to be encouraged to return to normal length after resistance training and stretch those that need length improved. Consider which position – standing, sitting or lying – would best suit the individual for each of these stretches. Examples of static standing, sitting and lying stretches are shown in figure 3.6 on pages 85–7. Finally, consider whether the stretch should be:

- active – opposing muscle is used to bring about the stretch, or;

- passive – external force (gravity or another part of the body) is used to bring about the stretch;

- static – the stretch is held still for 10 seconds to 2 minutes, or;

- dynamic – the exerciser is encouraged to move at the joint(s) the muscle crosses, through slow, controlled movement, taking the muscle through its greatest active range – usually repeated five to 10 times.

Figure 3.6 Examples of stretch positions

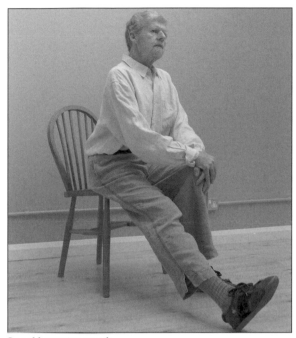

Seated hamstring stretch

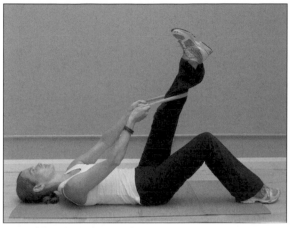

Assisted floor hamstring stretch

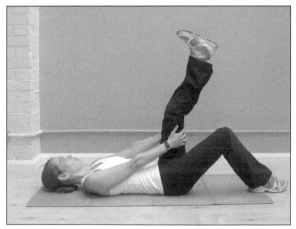

Floor hamstring stretch

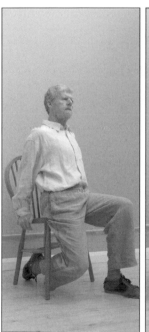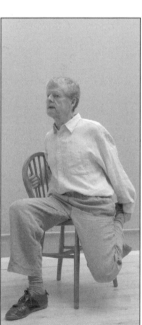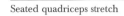

Seated quadriceps stretch

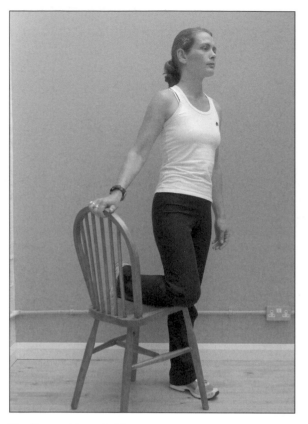

Standing quadriceps stretch

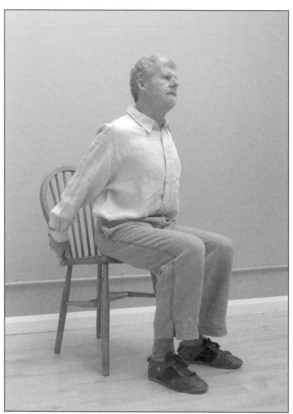

Seated chest stretch

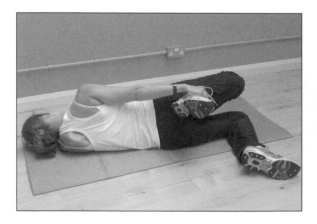

Floor quadriceps stretch

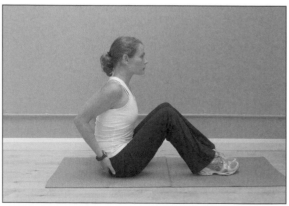

Floor chest stretch

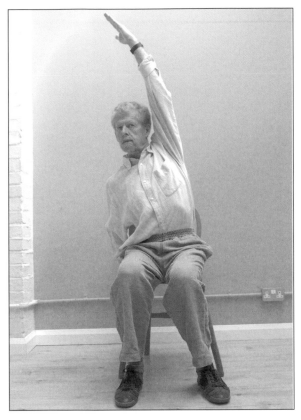

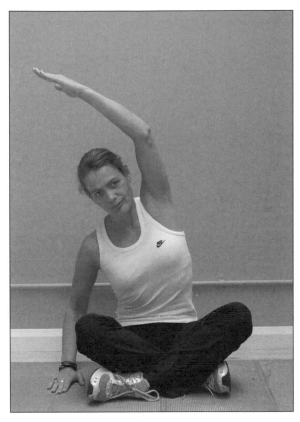

Seated/floor lats

At the end of the cool-down, if the individual would benefit from it and if there is a suitable environment, a relaxation element can be included. Within most gyms this does not work effectively, due to the volume of people and noise. However, where a studio or home environment is available, it may be possible to sit or lie comfortably and either rest or focus on breathing. Many relaxation techniques exist. Whichever works for each individual is the best to go with.

FUNCTIONAL EXERCISE TRAINING 15

The majority of disabled people who are interested in accessing fitness facilities are interested in improving their everyday life. More specifically, they are interested in improving their function to reduce the challenges they face in their everyday life. These challenges vary from individual to individual; at their most basic they include the physical abilities required to dress, wash, walk, work a wheelchair or eat independently. At their most advanced they include the return to sporting participation, up to the elite level, for those who have recently acquired an impairment.

When discussing an exercise programme with a person who finds everyday tasks difficult, they are unlikely to be motivated by hearing that the exercise in question is going to improve the strength or endurance of their triceps. They are much more likely to be sold by the idea that it will aid their ability to reach for things on high shelves, power their wheelchair, or scratch their back! In other words, when programming it is important to consider the way in which the client thinks about exercise, sometimes seeing it from a far less scientific perspective. Of course, the skill is then in combining the everyday language with the scientific background. When Newton discovered gravity he did so when the apple fell on his head. This is a fine example of how to combine the everyday with the scientific!

The value of each and every exercise within a programme should be known and linked to the requirements of each individual. Take time to examine the everyday actions your clients say are difficult, noting the muscle groups and movements involved. Attempt to replicate simpler or even more challenging versions of these actions within the exercise programme.

Actions can be made simpler by:
- performing on a stable surface;
- performing on a non-moving surface;
- using isolation (single-joint) exercises;
- using machines that limit movement selection.

Actions can be made more complex by:
- performing on an unstable surface, such as a stability ball;
- performing on a moving surface, such as a treadmill;
- using compound (multi-joint or multi-limb) exercises;
- using bodyweight, free weights or cables that allow complete self-selection of movement.

Figure 3.7 shows a classic route for complexity progression.

Figure 3.7 Complexity progression route

For a squat:

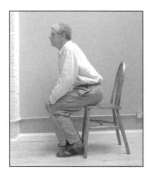

Sit to stand, hands on thighs for extra support (see above)

Sit to stand, hands on chair to start for slight extra support

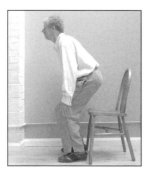

Sit to stand with hands by sides (see above)

Sit to stand with changes of mind on the way down

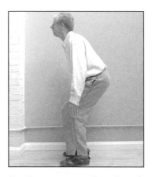

Small-range squats (see above)

Full-range squats

For a balance exercise:

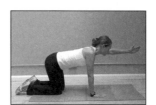

One arm

Isolation exercises, although simpler in terms of motor skills, often put greater stress on the body due to the total force having to go through one joint. Life usually involves moving more than one joint at a time. Although this is more complex in terms of motor skills, it spreads the load over a wider area.

While a stability ball undoubtedly increases complexity and encourages use of core muscles, for most people it is not life-related. The majority of my life does not involve me sitting or standing on an unstable surface. I sometimes stand up while on a bus ride and I very occasionally go waterskiing but these are the only exceptions. Consider for your clients the role of a stability ball within their exercise programme.

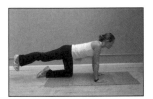

One leg

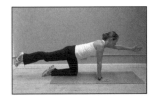

One arm and opposite leg – contralateral
(Note: the body generally chooses to work in diagonal planes)

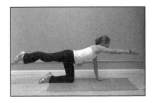

One arm and the leg on the same side – ipsilateral

Top tips for discovering new exercises

To improve knowledge and gain ideas about the range of exercises for each muscle, consider organising a workshop with work colleagues. Each person takes it in turn to demonstrate an exercise. Have available and use as varied a selection of equipment as possible. Such brainstorming sessions can often be very effective in developing lateral thinking, as they encourage experimentation.

CLOTHING, FOOTWEAR AND EQUIPMENT

16

Clothing and footwear

People should be given permission to participate in clothing in which they feel comfortable. Advice can be given to assist with comfort, such as encouraging women to wear trousers instead of, or in addition to, a skirt, in order to protect their decency. Some people may be interested in wearing clothing that helps them to fit in with others, but in most cases usual everyday clothing does not affect the health and safety of exercising.

Trainers, while allowing freedom of foot movement, are often highly cushioned, creating a trampoline-like effect when walking. Participants who find standing balance difficult will find that trainers can worsen this further. In such cases, advice should be given to find shoes that are relatively flat (some people find that a small heel assists their walking), have a flexible sole, are enclosed at the toe and have a strap around the back. The old style of trainers such as 'Green Flash' are ideal, but often the participant's usual footwear will suffice.

Equipment

There has been a belief that disabled people need specialist equipment in order to exercise. Research by the Gary Jelen Sports Foundation in 1999 found that poor design in fitness equipment was an important reason why disabled people were not participating in fitness activities. In 2000 there were only two suppliers interested in supplying equipment for use by disabled people, while in 2006 this number had climbed to a staggering 21! All the largest companies designing, manufacturing and selling fitness equipment in the world market are now committed to the supply of inclusive equipment.

It was originally assumed that major changes needed to be made to conventional equipment to make it useable by disabled people, but with the assistance of research by the IFI, it was realised that conventional equipment simply needed better design, with a more user-centred approach for all. In fact, with attention to matching instructor skills (communication, demonstration, and so on), planning and environmental factors to the needs of each participant, the importance of working with specialist equipment is dramatically reduced, as shown in figure 3.8 on page 94. This shows the cumulative benefit of all these factors.

A variety of adapted conventional or specialised fitness equipment can be seen in figure 3.9 on pages 94–5. Adaptations that make use of equipment easier for everyone, not just disabled people, can be said to be sense-able and body-centred. These include:

- colour contrast to prevent tripping over the equipment and for ease of locating adjustments;
- larger print for ease of reading instructions/information;
- seats that move out for use of equipment when standing or from a wheelchair;
- back supports for those who lack postural stability;
- strapping/wrapping to assist grip.

Figure 3.8 Dependence on equipment

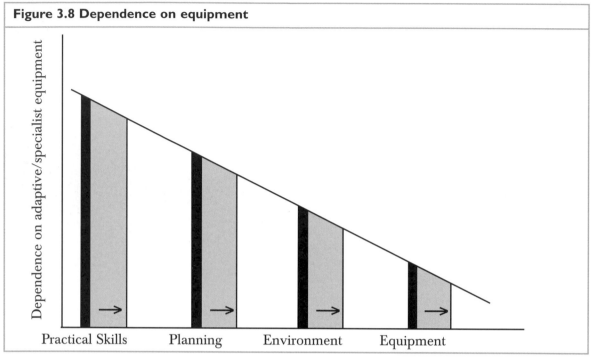

Adapted from Paul, S., *Equal Adventure*, 2005

Figure 3.9 Adapted fitness equipment

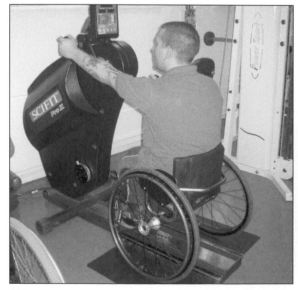

Arm ergometer

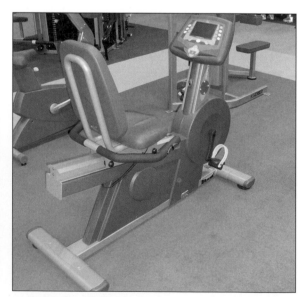

treadmill/bike with strips

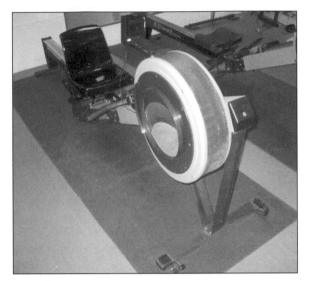

Adapted rower

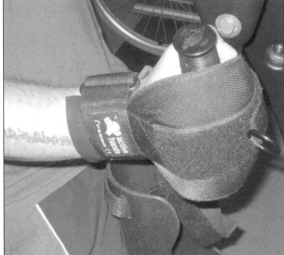

Strapping/wrapping for grip

Table 3.5	Small exercise equipment	
Equipment	**Benefits**	**Cautions**
Dumbbell	Small weight increments; Allows for independent use of each side of the body (unilateral movement); Allows for training of motor skills/functional for ADLs; Available in a variety of textures for ease of grip; Available with straps for assistance with grip; Available in bright colours for ease of sight and added fun; Easy to store; Relatively cheap to purchase.	Can be dropped, causing injury.
Barbell	Allows for training of motor skills/functional for ADLs; Allows for training of motor skills/functional for ADLs; Available in a variety of textures for ease of grip; Easy to store; Relatively cheap to purchase	Can be dropped, causing injury.

Ankle/wrist weight	Small weight increments; Allows for independent use of each side of the body (unilateral movement); Allows for training of motor skills/ functional for ADLs; No grip or hand function required; Available in bright colours for ease of sight and added fun; Easy to store; Relatively cheap to purchase.	Does not involve grip and therefore limits improvements in life-related lifting for those who have potential to grip.
Band	Non-threatening for those people unfamiliar with fitness equipment; Very low starting resistance available for the smallest muscle groups and the least fit people; Very small resistance increments possible for graduated progression; Allows for training of motor skills/ functional for ADLs; Encourages controlled movement, especially during the eccentric phase; Easy grip options; Available in bright colours for ease of sight and added fun; Very easy to store; Very cheap to purchase; Ideal for home use.	Need to be regularly checked for tears/holes and thrown away if there are any; People with a latex allergy should wear gloves when holding a band; Small risk of injury if the band snaps during use; Ensure band is gripped correctly without wrapping in such a way as to restrict blood flow (see fig. 3.10 on page 98); Lifespan of the band is extended by keeping it dry.
Tube	Non-threatening for those people unfamiliar with fitness equipment; Very low starting resistance available for the smallest muscle groups and the least fit people; Very small resistance increments possible for graduated progression; Allows for training of motor skills/ functional for ADLs; Encourages controlled movement,	Need to be regularly checked for tears/holes and thrown away if there are any; Lifespan of the tube is extended by keeping it dry.

	especially during the eccentric phase; Easy grip options; Available in bright colours for ease of sight and added fun; Very easy to store; Very cheap to purchase; Ideal for home use.	
Ball	Allows for training of co-ordination and grip strength; Available in different colours for ease of sight and added fun; Available in different sizes for ease of grip and different usage (e.g. throwing or sitting on); Available in different textures for ease of grip and different flight potential (e.g. a balloon versus a football); Sports-related; Easy to store; Very cheap to purchase.	Consider suitability of the environment for throwing and catching games; Balls for sitting on should be made of anti-burst material.
Stability disc	Allows for training of balance and motor skills; Can be inflated to any different level, for different abilities and for graduated progression; Available in different colours for ease of sight and added fun; Can be used for standing on or sitting on to increase challenge in other exercises, or can be used as a postural aid; Can be used for throwing, like a frisbee; Very easy to store; Very cheap to purchase.	Consider suitability of the environment for throwing and catching games.

In facilities that lack modern inclusive equipment, older conventional equipment may still work effectively, but the approach to its use may need adapting. As always, adaptation is the key.

Equipment layout can make a big difference to accessibility for all users. Modern facilities, keen to offer usage to as many members as possible during peak periods, tend to pack their gyms full of equipment, leaving little room for manoeuvre. While there should still be sufficient room for a wheelchair user to move around the resistance equipment, it is not necessary to have space between the same

Fig 3.10

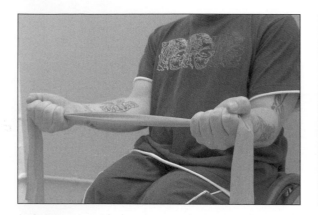 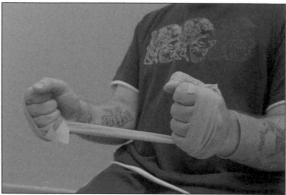

Resistance band grip: correct (*left*); incorrect (*right*)

pieces of equipment, such as between every treadmill or bike. Only one of each piece of equipment needs to have space beside it, such as the end treadmill in a row. If possible, a rowing machine should be placed with space to one side and a wall to the other, to act as a mobility aid when moving on to and up from the seat.

Where modular resistance equipment is inaccessible, small equipment provides a never-ending range of opportunities. Dumbbells, barbells, bands, tubes and balls are just some of such equipment. Table 3.5 shows the benefits and cautions for each of these.

In the home exercise market, where an individual is interested in purchasing equipment specific to their personalised needs, there is still a role for specialist equipment. In particular, there is a substantial range of equipment available that is ideal for purchase by wheelchair users, including pulley systems that can be reached by a seated person unable to reach as high as a standing person and passive leg machines (those that can be set to bring about movement in paralysed limbs).

Top tips for sign language communication

- Learn how to sign your name, using the alphabet shown in figure 3.11 on page 102
- Offer to learn a few useful signs from your clients
- Some people who use BSL will not be willing or able to speak and may wish to use a sign language interpreter. Local interpretation services can be found within the phone book or through the RNID
- Working with a sign language interpreter is much like working with any foreign language interpreter. You should speak directly to your client, pausing as required by the interpreter. Use the word 'you' rather than 'he' or 'she' when asking a question. Ensure you use the interpreter only for language interpretation, rather than for seeking information about the client.

In addition, follow the guidance for verbal communication and lip-reading (see page 100).

Sign Supported English

Sign Supported English tends to be used by people who have a significant hearing impairment. Using signs from BSL, it is used to enhance the spoken word. As with BSL, work with your clients to learn some signs that you both find helpful.

Deaf-Blind Sign Language

Deaf-Blind Sign Language is used by people who have both hearing and visual impairments. It involves signs being touched on to the palm. Again, locate an interpreter and work patiently with the client to develop a rapport.

Makaton

Makaton is a form of sign language used by people with learning disabilities who have difficulty with spoken language. It has a range of signs to assist with communicating needs and wants.

Some Makaton signs that could be useful within the fitness environment can be seen in figure 3.12 on page 103.

The teaching sequence

The teaching sequence commonly proposed in fitness training manuals (*see* fig. 3.13 on page 104) is based on the theory that individuals learn in different ways. If all these different ways are addressed, then it follows that everyone will receive the message.

People learn through one of, or a mix of, three different senses, these being sight, sound and touch, as shown in figure 3.14.

Task

Consider how each of these sensory learning styles is reflected in the teaching sequences mentioned above. Which of these represents your learning style? Now consider your friends and regular clients. Do you know their learning styles? Do you, your friends and clients have a mix of styles, rather than only one?

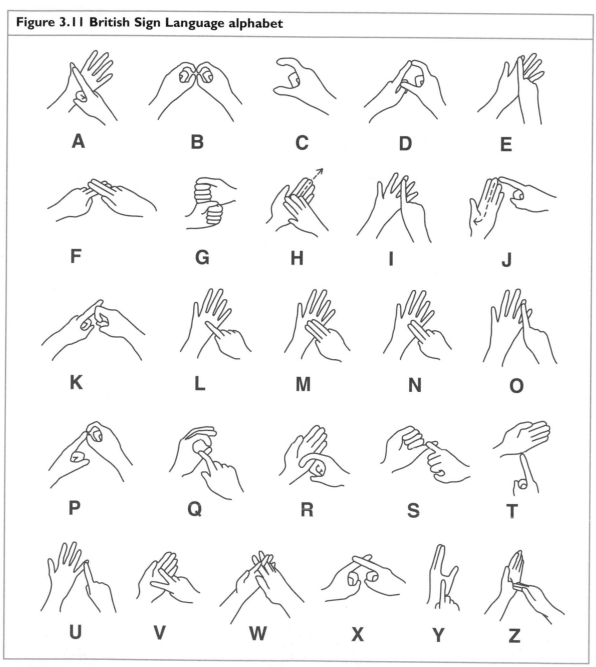

Figure 3.11 British Sign Language alphabet

Figure 3.12 Sample Makaton signs

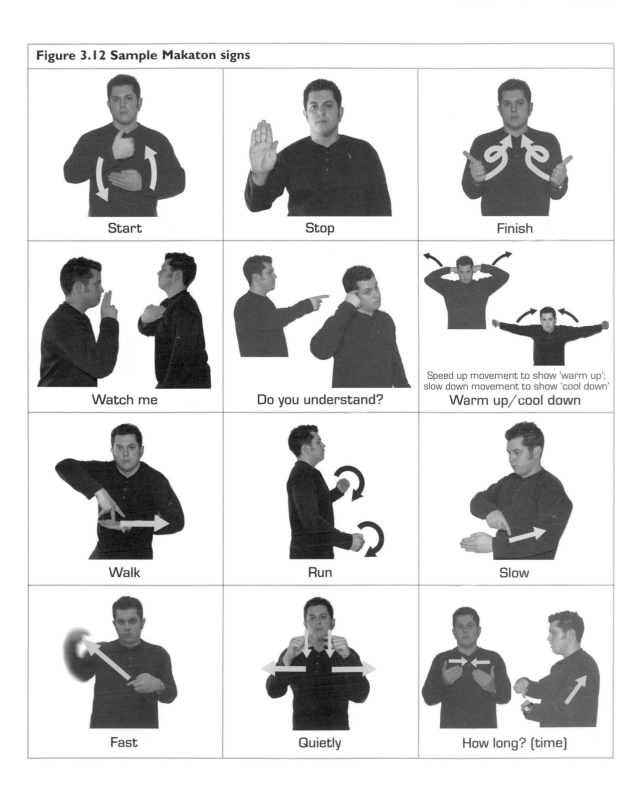

Start	Stop	Finish
Watch me	Do you understand?	Speed up movement to show 'warm up'; slow down movement to show 'cool down' **Warm up/cool down**
Walk	Run	Slow
Fast	Quietly	How long? (time)

Figure 3.13 The conventional teaching sequence

For cardiovascular exercises:
1 Name the exercise;
2 Demonstrate the exercise;
3 Explain key points about the exercise;
4 Let the client try the exercise;
5 Provide feedback to praise and correct.

For resistance exercises:
1 Name the exercise;
2 Name the muscles and identify where these are on the body;
3 Demonstrate the exercise;
4 Explain key points about the exercise;
5 Let the client try the exercise;
6 Provide feedback to praise and correct.

It is important to be mindful of how impairment might affect learning. Some disabled people will have a reduction or total loss in one or more of their senses; for example a blind person will have no use of sight, a deaf person will have no use of sound.

The reality of working with disabled people is that, for each individual, a different teaching sequence should be used. This is actually no different from effective work with non-disabled people. While some people will feel the need to observe a demonstration in order to be safe, others will want to get going at the first opportunity.

Case study

I was asked to work with a female with Down's Syndrome, aged 21, who was keen to use the gym. After successfully completing a pre-exercise assessment (PAR-Q and measures relating to her goals), I was ready to start introducing her new programme. The girl was full of energy and had full physical function. She listened carefully, but tended to forget quickly the information spoken. She initially observed well, but soon tended to look at anything and everything going on in the busy gym environment. She was also very keen to please, and tended to answer 'yes' to any question she was asked.

Her preferred learning style was found to be Kinaesthetic. I stood directly in front of her and asked her to copy (or shadow) my movements. I used my standing position to cut off her views of the surroundings, helping her to remain focussed. By shadowing all movements, I remained in control of speed, range of movement and number of repetitions, and was also easily able to reinforce the correct line of movement. The client was instantly able to interpret the information and relate it to her own technique.

Once your client starts exercising, ensure you offer feedback, either to praise or to correct. Continue providing feedback until the exercise is performed safely. You may have to move on before it is truly effective, but you must never compromise safety.

Wherever possible, within an exercise class or

Table 2.1	Correct and incorrect language use	
Visual (sight)	Auditory (sound)	Kinaesthetic (touch/feel)
Tendency to look up between sentences; Tendency to use words such as 'see' and to be descriptive in their talk; Tendency to recall memories by playing back a film;	Tendency to look across between sentences; Tendency to use words such as 'hear' or replace words with sounds; Tendency to recall memories by recalling sounds;	Tendency to look down between sentences; Tendency to use words such as 'feel' and to use hand gestures; Tendency to recall memories by recalling a sense of being there;
↓	↓	↓
Observation Demonstration	Speech Explanation	Getting involved Participation

the gym, you should be trying to encourage independence in exercise. When attempting to promote independence, consider how, from the very first session, you can use your skills to promote this independence. For example, after working on a one-to-one basis for a few sessions, you may be able to observe some parts of the exercise programme from a distance on subsequent sessions, before eventually only being required to assist in the set-up of specific exercises, or realising that you are now not required at all.

Consider the best use of any carers or assistants, as they may be able to learn about the exercise programme, to assist or take over responsibility for introducing, observing and correcting technique on each exercise.

Observation and feedback

Observation skills are extremely important. Without good observation and feedback, exercise can be unsafe and the exerciser is at risk of injury. Many will only feel safe in the fitness environment thanks to your knowledge and skills.

Consider the following when observing:

- Is it necessary to observe from different positions – at the front, sides and back of the individual?
- Would moving around to observe be uncomfortable for your client, causing them to lose balance or exercise technique?
- Would questioning the client aid your

observation and help in their understanding of exercise technique?
- Is it possible to select an exercising position that makes best use of the environment to enable use of mirrors and/or space to move around?

Relate back what you have observed to help the exerciser build a more in-depth picture of their exercise technique. Your feedback will ensure safety and enhance the effectiveness of each exercise. Feedback can be in the form of praise or correction, both of which can be motivating if phrased appropriately.

Meaningful praise is possibly the greatest instant motivation available. To not only be told you are doing something well, but why you are doing it well, is truly uplifting. It also helps for future sessions, when the individual is more likely to remember the correct technique.

Correction, given in a positive manner, can also be motivating. It is essential for injury avoidance and aids concentration as the exerciser processes the information and connects it into their movement.

The words and phrases you use when giving feedback should be reflective of the individual with whom you are speaking, so that they are both understood and motivating. For example, here is the same phrase stated in three different ways:
- Well done, you are keeping your arms straight;
- Good. Can you keep your elbows from bending?

- That's good. Now, as you lift the weight, try to lengthen your arms towards the side walls.

Touch protocol

Wherever possible, unless you have built up a rapport with an individual in a personal training setting, touch should be avoided. Always attempt to feed back using words, hand signals and demonstration. Some people will be offended by touch and others in the environment may believe it to be inappropriate. Allowing the individual to improve technique without hands-on guidance also improves their absorption of the technique for repeat performance in the future.

While some people may be able to hear, see, feel and understand, many who have poor body awareness or who have a condition affecting information-processing will find it difficult to transfer corrections into action.

If, having tried other avenues, you decide that touch is necessary, it is often possible to give control over touch to the exerciser. By placing your hand at the point you would like them to move to, they can move to touch you at that point or up close to it (*see* Fig. 3.15 on page 107). If you really feel the need to reposition or guide movement using a hands-on approach, ask the individual for permission to touch their hand/arm/foot before doing so. Warning that you are about to touch is important to ensure you maintain a professional approach.

Figure 3.15

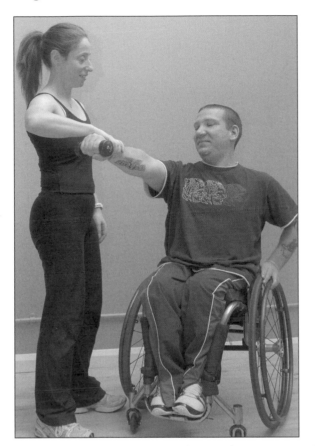 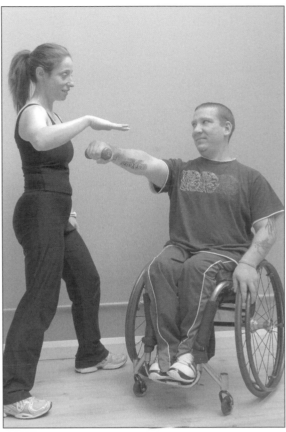

Touch protocol: incorrect approach (*left*); correct approach (*right*)

EXERCISE SELECTION

18

Introduction

Exercises for disabled people are in principle the same as exercises for non-disabled people. You may find that you need to be ready with alternative solutions when more conventional exercises are not suited to the individual, either because they cannot access the equipment or because their body is unsuited to the range of movement inherent in the exercise. There are many, many different ways of exercising muscles. The greater the repertoire of exercises you have knowledge about, the easier it will be for you to offer successful options.

No one book or website is able to offer *all* possibilities for every exercise. Be prepared to experiment with your clients, to find exercises that suit their personality and body, even if you have not previously seen the exercise in a text book or on a website. Check any new exercises with other colleagues if you are concerned over their safety.

Individuality

While some disabled people will be able to perform exercises as you would hope to see them in a book or on film, others will have differences in their body alignment that mean their range of movement and line of movement need adapting. If you were to take an image of their body in anatomical position, they would be unable to line up their arms, spine and/or legs (*see* Fig. 3.16 below).

Figure 3.16

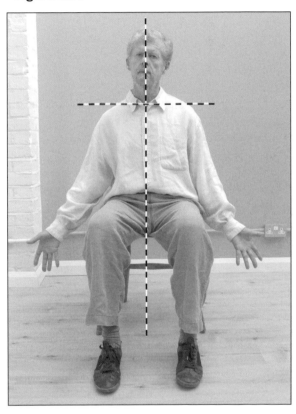

Vertical and horizontal lines highlight offset body alignment

It therefore follows that the line of movement will require adapting when exercising. In such cases you will need to reframe your image of how the exercise should be performed or how it should look, taking into account the individual's characteristics. For example, someone with osteoarthritis may have a misaligned knee, causing their squat technique to be asymmetrical; one leg (correctly) moving differently from the other. Be prepared to observe carefully, to ensure that any feedback given is appropriate to each individual's body alignment, ability and capability.

Posture

Posture has been defined as 'the arrangement of body parts in a state of balance' (Posture Committee of the American Academy of Orthopaedic Surgeons, 1947). Posture provides a frame of reference from which the individual can organise their own movements with relation to the external environment.

Correct posture creates:

- a solid foundation for all movements;
- optimal biomechanical efficiency for effortless pain-free movement;
- balance between the right and left sides and the front and back of the body;
- reduced risk of injury;
- reduced risk of degeneration of muscles and joints.

One way to think about posture is using the imagery of a tent. A tent is held secure and upright by tethering it with guy ropes, of even length and even tension. Should any one or more of these ropes be uneven in length or tension, the tent is at risk of falling down. The greater the wind factor and the less firm the ground is, the greater the risk of the tent falling. In the same way, as a person with poor posture starts to exercise, they are at increased risk of injury from the increasing amounts of stress put through their body by factors such as limb movement, increased resistance, or changes in standing surface.

Posture will vary according to the type of activity being performed:

- **Static** posture – alignment when the body is still (standing, sitting or lying).

- **Dynamic** posture – alignment when the body is moving (walking, running and lifting).

Optimal static posture should be set before commencing an exercise. Then, when an exercise is performed, it should be done with optimal dynamic posture. Just because static posture is optimal, it does not follow that dynamic posture will automatically be optimal.

For some disabled people who have joint deformities, optimal posture may not look as it does in this or any other book; it should be interpreted according to the individual's muscle and joint structure.

Figure 3.17 Correct seated posture

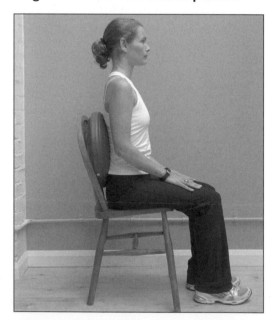

When exercising from a seated position, ideally sit to the front third of the chair to enable a stable base of support and to engage/train core stability muscles. Only use a chair back if essential. Use of equipment (such as that shown in fig 3.17) may be helpful for maintenance of optimal posture or to limit pain.

Figure 3.18 Correct standing posture

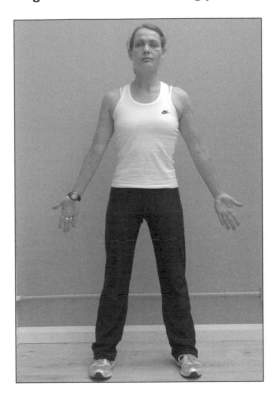

Getting down to and up from the floor: backward chaining

While some people will be able to get down to and up from the floor without any difficulty, for others this provides a real challenge. A fear of not being able to get up if having fallen sets off a vicious cycle; it causes people to become more sedentary, leading to further secondary conditions, a greater risk of falling and therefore an even greater fear of falling.

Any ambulant individual, for whom moving to/from the floor is difficult, should practise this as part of an exercise programme, whenever there are others around to support and assist. A helpful technique, known as backward chaining, is the approach often suggested. This requires use of a firm chair, or low table to act as a stability aid. As backward chaining is a relatively complex task, it may be necessary to break the whole task up into smaller tasks, gradually linking these together as ability progresses.

Figure 3.19 Backward chaining

Part A:
1 Step forwards with the strongest leg;
2 Place hand on chair (see below);

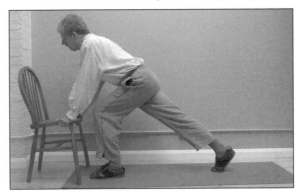

3 Ensure weight is over chair, shoulders above wrists;
4 Step back leg through, maintaining slightly bent knees;
5 Transfer hands to thighs and walk hands up thighs until standing.

Part B:
1 As Part A 1–3;
2 Slide leg backwards until there is sufficient space between the two feet to accommodate the back knee;
3 Lower the back knee within a pain-free range (see below);
4 As Part A 4–5.

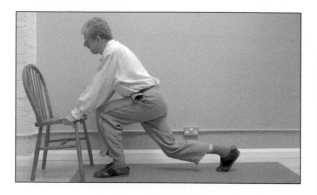

Part C:
1 As Part B 1–3;
2 Lower the back knee to the floor and release the toes (see below);

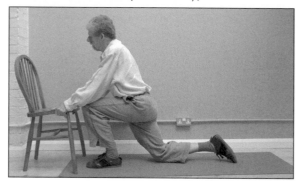

3 Lower the front knee to the floor (see below);

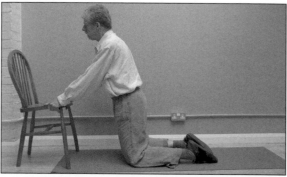

4 Lower hands to the floor and crawl back away from chair (see below).

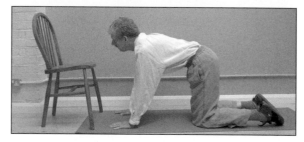

To get back up:
1 Bring the strongest leg through until the foot is firmly on the floor;
2 Place both hands firmly on the chair;
3 Push through the arms and the front leg until standing with slightly bent knees;
4 Transfer hands to thighs and walk hands up thighs until standing.

SPECIFIC MEDICAL CONDITIONS

19

Specific medical conditions require specific programming and instruction skills. This section provides advice for a range of medical conditions.

Advice is given based on each single medical condition, but it is not uncommon for individuals to have several medical conditions at the same time. Therefore, all the advice on each medical condition should be gathered together and checked to ensure no one piece of advice opposes another. If this is the case, the most important rule is to programme exercise that does not cause increased pain, nor risks new injury or illness. An example of this is given in the case study below.

Case Study

A 68-year-old woman attended the gym for a new exercise programme, following a suggestion from her GP. She had osteoarthritis in her left knee and hip, and had also been diagnosed with low-grade osteoporosis. Her GP had suggested that exercise might prevent these worsening.

Resistance training guidelines for these conditions are at odds, as follows:

- Osteoarthritis – low resistance, low repetitions, not to fatigue to improve joint stability but avoid increased inflammation;
- Osteoporosis – high resistance, low repetitions strength training to fatigue, to load the bones.

Since no exercise programme should be causing new pain or increasing injury risk, the guidelines for osteoarthritis were used in the muscles crossing the affected joints, but those for osteoporosis were used in all other muscles.

Orthopaedic conditions

Orthopaedic conditions are those that affect the bones and/or the way they function/articulate, that is to say, the joints.

1 Name of condition

Arthritis

2 Definition and incidence of condition

There are over 200 different forms of arthritis. The two most common groups are osteoarthritis and rheumatoid arthritis.

- osteo = bone
- rheum = blood
- arthro = joint
- itis = inflammation

Osteoarthritis is a degenerative 'wear and tear' disease that occurs at one or more localised joints – usually those joints that get repeated use in loading, including knees, hips and spine. In people using loaded hand movements, such as was typical with use of old typewriters, it may appear in the hands. It is most common in older adults.

Rheumatoid arthritis is an auto-immune inflammatory disease that occurs when the body attacks its own tissue – most commonly the tissue at the joints, but also in internal organs. It is more common in women than in men and is usually first diagnosed in people aged between 20 and 40.

There are estimated to be nine million people living with an arthritic condition in the UK; five million with osteoarthritis and 387,000 with rheumatoid arthritis.

3 Main characteristics of the condition

Osteoarthritis may affect only one joint or it may affect many. It starts with destruction of the cartilage at the bone ends, followed by the development of bony protrusions (osteophytes) where the bone ends rub against each other. This creates inflammation, pain and stiffness at the joint and often wastage in surrounding muscle tissue.

In rheumatoid arthritis, destruction of the synovial membrane causes drying up of the joints, which deform and misalign over time. Chronic pain is worsened after remaining in one position for a long time, such as after sleeping. Pain and the ability to move are often worst in the mornings. Inflammatory flare-ups are characteristic, during which the joints are so inflamed that any movement becomes extremely difficult and painful.

Due to the level of pain, many people with these conditions become sedentary.

4 Effects of the condition on exercise response

Degenerative and inflammatory joint diseases have the same impact upon exercise. In those joints affected, range of movement will be inhibited and there will be a loss of ability to perform rapid or repetitive movements.

Movements involving impact are likely to increase pain.

Muscular tone is decreased around the joint(s), causing a loss in muscular strength. Pain increases the level of energy expenditure involved in any movement. Where joints are misaligned, textbook body positions and text-book movements are no longer possible.

5 Medications and their effect on exercise response

Anti-inflammatory medications can noticeably benefit exercise. Liaise with the client's prescribing practitioner to ask whether it would be advisable to take an anti-inflammatory medication 30 minutes before commencing exercise.

Exercise, other than mobility, should be avoided for one week following injections into the joint. Long-term use of steroids can increase the risk of osteoporosis.

6 Important rules

- Avoid morning exercise – wait until joint stiffness has decreased
- Never exercise during an acute flare-up
- Never exercise through increasing levels of pain
- Monitor pain with a pain scale as well as monitoring exercise intensity, as pain may prevent ideal exercise intensity
- Unaffected joints should be exercised as for any other healthy adult
- Introduce only one new exercise per affected joint per session. If there is an inflammatory response later the same day or the next day, it is then easy to identify the cause
- If grip is affected, be prepared to offer different grip surfaces or strapping/wrapping solutions (*see* fig. 3.20 on page 115).

Figure 3.20

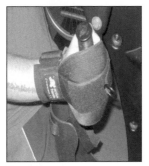

Strapping

7 Goals of the exercise programme

- Improve joint integrity – stability and function
- Manage pain
- Improve energy levels
- Improve mood
- Prevent secondary diseases caused by lack of physical activity.

8 Programming principles

Some people will find training in a swimming pool is most successful, for example in an aqua class. The pool temperature should be set slightly higher than usual.

Warm-up

Start with mobilisation of affected joints, without increasing pain levels, initially through small ranges of movement. For joints in the leg and spine this should be performed from a seated, non-weight-bearing position.

Consider seated (non-weight-bearing) options for pulse-raising activities, especially if standing balance is poor. The seat position on the bike may need to be set relatively close, to accommodate restricted knee or hip mobility. It may be possible to take the seat back once any affected joints have been mobilised.

Repetitive movements can increase inflammation, so a variety of small-range movements may be needed for effective pulse-raising.

Seated stretches may be helpful for body awareness, but should be entered into slowly and only once the muscles are truly warm.

CV

As with warm-up, consider small-range movements. Duration may be limited due to an inflammatory response. If possible, use joints unaffected by arthritis, so as to increase the pulse rate higher and for longer.

RESISTANCE

Some resistance machines will force misaligned joints through unsuitable planes of movement and therefore should be avoided. Pulleys and small equipment can be useful.

Perform only one repetition, with a low resistance, through small range on the first occasion. If there is no negative response, increase repetitions, range and lastly resistance over the following sessions. Note that for life-related benefits, the ability to perform over a greater range can be the most helpful gain.

Co-ordination

Consider whether improvements in gait should be worked on during the CV component.

Cool-down and flexibility

Developmental stretches should be avoided in affected joints. Only perform static, maintenance stretches. Consider which stretch position would be the most comfortable. Often seated stretches provide the best option.

9 Teaching principles

If the exerciser has difficulty with cervical spine rotation, ensure you are standing directly in front when engaging in conversation.

Feed back on differences you notice in range of movement between the two sides of the body to improve body awareness. Note that it may be in the client's best interests to maintain these differences.

10 Personalise it!

Provide guidance related, for example, to the client's other medical conditions; goals; likes and dislikes; lifestyle.

---

1 Name of condition

Osteoporosis

2 Definition and incidence of condition

'Osteo' means 'bone' and 'porosis' means 'porous' (with pores/holes). Osteoporosis involves a progressive loss of bone strength and bone mineral density above the age-related norm. There are two types:

- Type I affects mainly women, is caused by oestrogen deficiency and usually occurs following the menopause;
- Type II affects men and women, usually over the age of 70 years, and is caused by vitamin D deficiency.

While osteoporosis may be a primary condition it is also a common secondary condition, for example due to long-term use of certain medications, spinal cord injury, or lack of physical activity resulting from another condition.

Fractures likely to be caused by osteoporosis occur in one in two women and one in five men over the age of 50.

3 Main characteristics of the condition

Osteoporosis causes a weakened skeleton that is prone to fractures, especially in the spine, hip and wrist. There is also a tendency to kyphotic posture ('dowager's hump'), causing:

- loss of standing balance;
- increased fear of falling;
- increased risk of falling;
- loss of neck mobility required for activities of daily life;
- loss of ability to expand the thorax for breathing.

Also characteristic are a loss of height, and pain.

4 Effects of the condition on exercise response

- Spine deformity can affect ventilatory capacity (the ability to breathe)
- Spine deformity and loss of spine mobility diminishes the field of vision and therefore affects communication
- Fear and risk of falling
- Fear and risk of further fractures
- Increased energy expenditure
- Low confidence and high anxiety.

5 Medications and their effect on exercise response

Some medications may cause bone pain, which usually disappears, but generally have no effect on exercise response. Often medication is in the form of vitamin and mineral supplementation.

6 Important rules

- Never perform exercises that load a flexed spine, for example abdominal curls, which have been shown to increase the risk of spinal fracture by up to 89 per cent – a greater risk than doing no exercise at all!
- Perform static abdominal exercises when standing, sitting or lying
- Improve standing balance by including exercises performed from a standing position, with a stability aid (chair, exercise machine) close by
- Avoid exercises that over-challenge standing balance (treadmill, stepper, cross-trainer)
- Perform strength-biased resistance training exercises at fracture risk sites
- Monitor movement between exercises as well as exercise technique.

7 Goals of the exercise programme

- Maintain and increase bone density
- Improve confidence in daily activities
- Improve mood
- Prevent secondary diseases caused by lack of physical activity.

8 Programming principles

Warm-up

As for any individual who has a tendency to a sedentary lifestyle, this should be long and gradual (*see* pages 71–83). Stretches should be performed in a stable, seated position to improve body awareness and encourage increased range of movement throughout the rest of the workout.

CV

Increase duration before intensity. Use any exercise that does not adversely affect posture or cause pain or discomfort. In pre-menopausal women and in men, include impact exercises.

Vary the force put through bone and muscle by changing the mode of exercise (or the gradient of walking) at least every 10 minutes.

Resistance

Work towards three sets at 80 per cent of 1RM, the equivalent to 8RM. Hold at peak strain for up to three seconds. Repeat at least three times per week.

Include exercises for muscles that cross the hip (quadriceps, hamstrings, abductors, adductors), spine (erector spinae, trapezius, transversus abdominis) and wrist (any exercise involving grip).

Balance

Include standing balance exercises, with appropriate, progressive levels of challenge. Include backward chaining (*see* fig. 3.19 on pages 111–2) to increase confidence and ability in getting up from the floor. Include floor-based activities once backward chaining is achievable, to improve confidence and mobility on the floor.

Cool-down and flexibility

Ensure a long and gradual cool-down, as above. Encourage comfortable static, developmental stretching to improve the range of movement and posture. Consider the best position for each stretch, remembering that it may not be possible to include floor-based options until the person is confident in their ability to get up from the floor. Encourage a daily stretch routine.

9 Teaching principles

If the individual has a reduced field of vision, stand directly in front whenever communicating.

10 Personalise it!

Provide guidance related, for example, to the client's other medical conditions: goals; likes and dislikes; lifestyle.

---

1 Name of condition

Limb amputation

2 Definition and incidence of condition

Limb amputation refers to the loss of one or more limbs as a result of another medical condition, trauma, tumour or congenital deformity. There are estimated to be more than 40,500 amputees in the UK population.

3 Main characteristics of the condition

Limb amputation is often a secondary condition, arising as a result of a primary condition. If the loss is due to another medical condition (commonly cardiovascular disease), characteristics of that condition should be taken into consideration.

The person may experience phantom pain – that is to say, pain in an area of the body that has been amputated. They may use a prosthetic limb and/or walking aids.

4 Effects of the condition on exercise response

Maximal heart rate will be reduced proportionate to the reduced volume of muscle mass. There is increased energy expenditure in walking related to the level of amputation: the higher the amputation, the greater the energy expenditure.

Posture is likely to be affected by the loss of bone and muscle. The greater the amount of weight loss, the greater the imbalance, and so the greater the effect on posture. Standing balance may be limited by above-knee leg amputation.

Any increase in physical activity will put increased stress on the stump of a leg amputation. This can cause skin intolerance (soreness through to infection) and/or pain in the stump. These symptoms can be further exacerbated by a badly fitting prosthesis or a heavy prosthesis. If the client changes weight, they should check the fitting. Keen sportspeople will invest in lightweight prostheses costing several thousand pounds.

5 Medications and their effect on exercise response

Medications are likely to be for the primary condition. Cardiovascular medications often have important effects on exercise response, including preventing the heart rate from rising proportionately to the intensity of exercise. Medications for phantom pain can cause drowsiness.

6 Important rules

- Assess the suitability of prosthetic limbs and walking aids
- Ensure that physical activity levels are increased gradually to avoid injury to a

stump, especially activities that load through the stump

- Although standing balance exercises are likely to improve standing balance for leg amputees, improvements may be limited by the prosthetic limb
- Check seated balance, which may be affected by loss of an arm or leg.

7 Goals of the exercise programme

- Improve confidence and function in ADLs, including walking
- Prevent muscular pain caused by muscle imbalance
- Manage weight, especially for high-level amputees with a significant loss of muscle mass
- Prevent secondary diseases caused by lack of physical activity.

8 Programming principles

Warm-up

As for any non-disabled person, this should be related to fitness level, with extra consideration for stability when exercising.

CV

Focus on the largest muscle groups available, in order to effectively raise the heart rate.

Resistance

Check stability when exercising from a standing and a seated position. For exercises that put force through the stump, ensure the resistance selected increases gradually over time, to allow adaptation of the tissue at the end of the stump.

Attempt to maintain, or increase, muscle mass in the area above an amputated limb. Use looped attachments available on the cable machine, strapped weights or looped resistance bands, being careful to ensure there is appropriate padding as required.

Co-ordination

Standing and seated balance and posture may not improve to full function, but should be targeted where there is a high-level amputation.

Cool-down and flexibility

As for any non-disabled person, the cool-down should be related to fitness level. Lying options are advisable for stretching the unaffected leg of a single-leg amputee.

9 Teaching principles

As for non-disabled people.

10 Personalise it!

Provide guidance related, for example, to the client's other medical conditions; goals; likes and dislikes; lifestyle.

Neurological conditions

Neurological conditions are those that are caused by a breakdown in one or more parts of the nervous system. The exact loss of function that results is dependent on the part(s) of the nervous system affected and, in progressive diseases, on the the stage of the disease. The nervous system is responsible for sending messages:

- within the brain (thoughts, emotions);
- from the brain to the body (movements);

- from the body to the brain (senses of smell, taste, touch).

---

1 Name of condition

Spinal cord injury

2 Definition and incidence of condition

This involves a partial or complete break of the spinal cord, causing loss of function below the site of the break. There are two types:

- *Tetraplegia* refers to damage between the cervical vertebrae and the top thoracic vertebra, causing impaired function of arms, legs, trunk and pelvic organs.
- *Paraplegia* refers to damage between the second and lowest thoracic vertebrae causing impaired function of legs, trunk and/or pelvic organs.

There could also be a loss of function due to damage to the lumbar or sacral vertebrae.

There are estimated to be 330,000 people living with a spinal cord injury in Europe. Most admissions into spinal injuries units are for people aged under 30, and 80 per cent are male.

3 Main characteristics of the condition

The level and completeness of the break will determine the loss of function, which could fall into one or more of three areas:

- Motor function – the ability to bring about voluntary movements, including control of bowel and bladder;
- Sensory function – the ability to feel sensation;
- Sympathetic nervous system – involuntary responses and reflexes.

There is an extremely high risk of developing secondary conditions, including:

- Metabolic syndrome – this involves one or more of obesity, hypertension, insulin resistance, low glucose tolerance, low levels of high-density lipoprotein ('good' cholesterol), poor make-up of low-density lipoprotein ('bad' cholesterol);
- Osteoporosis;
- Hypertension or hypotension.

4 Effects of the condition on exercise response

- A reduced ability to perform movements of the legs, trunk and/or arms
- A reduced ability to sustain high-intensity cardiovascular work
- A reduced ability to balance
- Poor thermoregulation
- Poor dilation and constriction properties in affected areas, causing blood-pooling and hypotension
- Autonomic dysreflexia – with injury above T6 (sixth thoracic vertebra of the spine) – in which the autonomic nervous system is overstimulated, causing sudden hypertension
- Pressure sores from sitting in one position for too long
- Overuse syndromes in arm muscles
- Early fatigue.

5 Medications and their effect on exercise response

Medications may cause hypotension and may increase urinary frequency

Support stockings and abdominal binders may help maintain blood pressure

6 Important rules

- Some wheelchair users will have some use of leg muscles. Find out the situation with your client to ensure the programme reflects their abilities
- Find out if the person would like to remain sitting in their wheelchair, or would prefer to transfer during the exercise session
- Ensure there is sufficient room for movement of the wheelchair around the exercising area
- Discourage sitting for long periods on hard surfaces. Encourage use of the wheelchair cushion if transferring to another chair
- Do not perform assisted stretches on paralysed muscles, as there is a risk of tearing them. Leave this to the spinally injured person or a trained specialist
- Ensure the exercising area is cool
- Encourage rehydration

7 Goals of the exercise programme

- Improve ADLs
- Maintain or improve independence
- Improve confidence and mood
- Manage weight
- Prevent secondary diseases caused by lack of physical activity

8 Programming principles

Warm-up

Offer an extended pulse-raiser to anyone who has a reduced ability to redistribute blood. Ensure all joints that function are effectively mobilised.

Consider the value of any stretching (*see* page 76).

CV

Most conventional CV machines focus on working the leg muscles. If these muscles cannot be used, focus on working the largest upper-body muscle groups, namely trapezius, latissimus dorsi and pectoralis. Adapt the rowing machine (*see* fig. 3.9 on pages 94–5), or perform lots of repetitions of low resistance exercises. Some gyms have arm ergometers that allow for flowing movement of the upper body.

Due to the reduced circulation in paralysed limbs, use of conventional heart rate percentage zones may not work. Depending on the level of function, maximal heart rate could be reduced by as much as 65 per cent. Be prepared to re-set heart rate goals, or use RPE scales for effective intensity monitoring.

Ensure heart rate is raised and lowered gradually to avoid unwanted changes in blood pressure and autonomic dysreflexia. Ensure there are opportunities for rehydration.

Within aerobics-style classes, note that sideways movement is impossible in a wheelchair. Apply a holding pattern to sidestepping/grapevines to allow wheelchair users time to turn. Also note that all changes of direction take more time, so holding patterns should also be used when changing from forward to backward movement.

Within circuit-style classes, note that a wheelchair user may move faster than someone who is walking/jogging.

Resistance

Consider using pulleys, bands and dumbbells for resistance training, especially where machines are inaccessible. Ensure the person and their wheelchair are stable when performing loaded activities. Movements above the head can cause the chair to fall backwards. A wheelchair is most stable when forces are applied sideways (wheel to wheel) rather than front to back. With this in mind, consider how to position the exerciser when performing loaded activities (*see* fig. 3.21). Similarly, if the exerciser lacks stability, encourage holding the side of the chair or a wheel. Consider the person's sitting position in the chair and whether to offer trunk support.

Be careful not to overload the small upper-body muscles, especially those used to stabilise the scapulae. Consider the order of exercises, looking at those that involve pulling, those that involve pushing, movements at shoulder level or above and movements below shoulder level.

Co-ordination

Some wheelchair users will value practising wheelchair skills. Sports hall lines and cones can be used to mark out challenging courses.

Figure 3.21

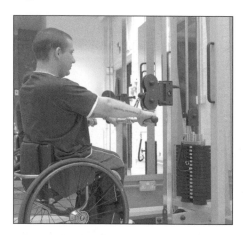
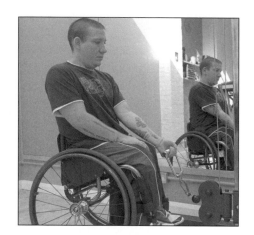

Incorrect position for loaded activities – front-on position

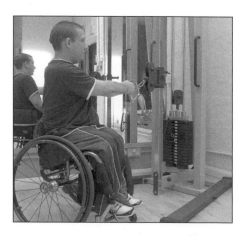
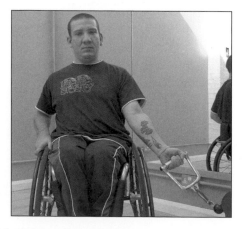

Correct position for loaded activities – side-on position

Cool-down and flexibility

Since the ability to redistribute blood can be poor, consider an extended cool-down. Stretch positions must be suitable to the individual's ability to move away from their chair and their ability to remain stable while seated.

9 Teaching principles

Attempt to sit down while talking to a wheelchair user so that you can gain eye contact at a similar level. Note that most gyms are full of spare seats on the exercise equipment!

10 Personalise it!

Provide guidance related, for example, to the client's other medical conditions: goals; likes and dislikes; lifestyle.

1 Name of condition

Stroke / Cerebrovascular accident (CVA)

2 Definition and incidence of condition

This conditions involves cell death caused by a loss of oxygen to part of the brain, due to a blood clot or a bleed in the vascular system supplying blood to that area of the brain.

Stroke is the third largest cause of death in the UK (after coronary heart disease and cancer). More than 130,000 people have strokes per year and there are estimated to be over 250,000 people living with impairments caused by stroke.

3 Main characteristics of the condition

The condition is characterised by one or more of the following:

- Impairment to sensory (touch/proprioception) and/or motor (movement) function on the opposite side of the body to the side of the brain where the stroke occurred. Motor problems usually initially cause weakness, with increased tone then following;
- Visual impairment and/or perception;
- Speech difficulties, including comprehension and word recognition;
- Confusion;
- Low mood/depression;
- Emotional changes, including laughing or crying for unknown reason.

There are commonly co-existing conditions such as high blood pressure or diabetes. The risk factor for having a stroke increases after having had one of these conditions.

4 Effects of the condition on exercise response

Motor problems mean muscles may be hypotonic (too little tension) or, less commonly, hypertonic/spastic (too much tension), causing grip difficulties and problems performing voluntary movement. Some people find it hard to co-ordinate certain planes of movement.

There may be difficulty with performing tasks in their correct sequence (dyspraxia) and standing balance and/or gait are often affected. In addition, processing of information given by the instructor may take longer. Short-term memory may be poor, causing the person to forget exercises from one session to the next. Motivation to exercise may vary and the person may experience early fatigue due to physical effort and mental concentration.

5 Medications and their effect on exercise response

Antihypertensive, anticonvulsant and antihypertonia medications are commonly prescribed. These may have the following side-effects:

- Prevent the heart rate from increasing in relation to the level of activity. RPE should be used instead of pulse-rate monitoring in such cases;
- Increase the likelihood of a hypotensive response to exercise, meaning warm-ups and cool-downs should be longer and more gradual;
- Increased bleeding after a cut;
- Low concentration;
- Drowsiness.

6 Important rules

- Never force muscles that are hypotonic
- Exercising in a standing position is less likely to set off muscle contractures
- If it is possible, place a short tennis ball into a spastic hand and leave it there while continuing with the workout. This seems to encourage the hand muscles to relax
- Be prepared to use wrappings and strappings to assist with securing grip and/or feet in foot pedals, noting that sudden release from these may be necessary
- Take note of any co-existing medical conditions
- Work to fatigue but never to failure
- Monitor movement between exercises, as well as technique while exercising.

7 Goals of the exercise programme

- Hasten recovery from the effects of the stroke (note that improvements may continue to be made for years after having a stroke)
- Reduce the risk of having another stroke
- Prevent secondary diseases caused by lack of physical activity
- Maintain independence
- Improve mood

8 Programming principles

Warm-up

Use a long warm-up, alternating pulse-raising with mobility to avoid early fatigue. Consider seated options if standing balance is poor.

CV

Include gait training if this is poor. Start with walking across the floor before introducing the added motor skills inherent with using a treadmill.

Work on increasing duration before intensity. Monitor fatigue (through observation and questioning) as well as exercise intensity.

Resistance

There is no evidence to suggest that resistance training increases spasticity. Since their strength abilities are likely to be asymmetrical, consider using different resistance levels on the two sides. Perform with the stronger side first, to enable the weaker side to learn movement quality.

Start with bodyweight-only exercises on weakened muscles. Consider using the functioning arm to support or assist the weak arm if required. Work on range of movement, before repetitions and before resistance.

The ability to grip will affect the type of equipment used. Include backward chaining if there is a difficulty in getting to the floor (see fig. 3.19 on pages 111–2). Resistance machines may be inappropriate if joints are misaligned. Use small equipment instead (*see* table 3.5 on pages 95–7).

Co-ordination

Where there is initial confusion or difficulty in sequencing activity, ensure task complexity progresses appropriately. It is important to train co-ordination for life-related activities. For example, relatively simple tasks such as throwing and catching a rubber ball can offer a fun, effective method of improving co-ordination when started as a small, single-joint movement not involving the ball and progressed through to the use of two balls at the same time.

Cool-down and flexibility

Offer a long cool-down as there may be a poor ability to return to the pre-exercise state. If standing balance and ability to get to the floor are poor, offer chair-based stretches (*see* fig. 3.6 on pages 85–7).

9 Teaching principles

Extra patience may be required, especially if there are sudden changes in mood, or difficulties with motivation or communication. Be prepared to explain exercises using very simple language and to repeat yourself if there is confusion or short-term memory has been affected.

10 Personalise it!

Provide guidance related, for example, to the client's other medical conditions: goals; likes and dislikes; lifestyle.

1 Name of condition

Multiple sclerosis (MS)

2 Definition and incidence of condition

'Multiple' means 'occurring in many sites' and 'sclerosis' means 'hard'. *Multiple sclerosis* is an autoimmune disease (where the body attacks itself), causing loss of the myelin sheath that insulates and protects nerve fibres from damage. This affects the rapid, smooth conduction of nerve impulses in the central nervous system, between the brain and the body. The cause is unknown, but is likely to be a mix of genetic and environmental factors.

There are three different types of MS:

- Relapsing remitting, characterised by relapses (worsening of symptoms) and remittance (reduction in or complete loss of symptoms) of unknown duration and severity;
- Secondary progressive, characterised by gradual worsening;
- Primary progressive, also characterised by gradual worsening.

Women are twice as likely as men to acquire MS, with first diagnosis generally between the ages of 20 and 40. There are estimated to be 85,000 people living with MS in the UK.

3 Main characteristics of the condition

Each individual tends to experience different symptoms, with a different degree of severity and in a different time and order of onset. Periods of relapse and remittance vary from a few days to several years, though progressive loss of function is usually found in areas that experience relapse on more than one occasion. Symptoms include:

- paralysis or paresis (partial paralysis);
- muscle spasm or stiffness;
- sensory loss (touch, proprioception, eyesight);

- numbness or tingling in the extremities (fingers and toes);
- cardio-acceleration and reduced blood pressure response;
- fatigue;
- heat sensitivity and loss of sweating mechanisms;
- poor concentration and memory;
- bladder and bowel problems (storage and emptying of waste);
- pain;
- depression.

4 Effects of the condition on exercise response

- Difficulty in controlling and co-ordinating movement
- Difficulty with standing balance
- Unusually fast heart rate response
- Decreased ability to thermo-regulate (control body temperature)
- Difficulty concentrating, working with RPE scales and remembering exercise technique
- Early fatigue that can worsen symptoms in relapse or cause onset of relapse
- Need to go to the toilet urgently

5 Medications and their effect on exercise response

There are four disease-modifying drugs available that can reduce the frequency and severity of relapses in some forms of MS. Side-effects can be severe, can worsen over time and include muscle ache, lethargy, depression and weight loss. Other drugs include muscle relaxants, with common side-effects being depression, drowsiness and muscle weakness.

6 Important rules

- Ensure the environment is cool and there are opportunities to rehydrate at regular intervals
- Most people prefer to exercise in the morning
- Suggest using the toilet before commencing exercise
- Be aware of trip hazards in those with a visual impairment
- Ensure regular monitoring of fatigue throughout. On days where fatigue is high before commencing, there should be no exercise but only relaxation. Consider having two programmes available, selecting the one most suitable related to energy levels on that day
- Ensure pulse is raised and lowered gradually to minimise cardio-acceleration and adverse blood pressure response
- Avoid or stop exercises that cause an increase in pain
- Find ways of assisting with exercise intensity monitoring using adapted RPE scales (*see* table 3.2 on page 69)
- Find ways of assisting with exercise memory, for example by using drawings with stick people
- Do not perform assisted stretches on paralysed muscles unless you have received specific training

7 Goals of the exercise programme

- Delay in the impact of the condition on everyday life function
- Improvement or maintenance in function, including standing balance – control of selected movement and range of movement
- Maintenance or improvement in muscle mass

- Improvement in mood
- Prevention of secondary diseases caused by lack of physical activity

8 Programming principles

Warm-up

Use this as an opportunity to assess the individual's abilities at each exercise session, including their level of fatigue, mood and level of motivation, range and control of voluntary movement. Offer an extended pulse-raiser to avoid undesired cardio-acceleration and a sudden fall in blood pressure.

Consider whether stretching is required, stretching those muscles that are shortened and spastic muscles that respond positively (that is, relax from spasm).

CV

Ensure this achieves very gradual pulse-raising and pulse-lowering. Include active rest periods, rather than long maintenance sections. Monitor fatigue carefully and also monitor temperature to ensure overheating is not occurring.

Have pedal clips or straps available for securing foot position on bikes.

Resistance

Select life-related/functional exercises involving muscular strength, muscular endurance and co-ordination. Consider using resistance exercises as active rests between CV exercises. Where one side is affected more than the other, perform exercises unilaterally, starting with a set on the least affected side.

Flexibility and Relaxation

Offer extended flexibility and relaxation components, finding a quiet environment for these wherever possible. Ensure different stretch positions are offered to improve comfort.

9 Teaching principles

Exercise should be used to aid motivation and therefore it should always entail success. Be prepared to repeat information, allow extra time for processing of information or find different ways to communicate it (verbally, in writing, using pictures or symbols).

10 Personalise it!

Provide guidance related, for example, to the client's other medical conditions: goals; likes and dislikes; lifestyle.

---

1 Name of condition

Parkinson's Disease

2 Definition and incidence of condition

Idiopathic Parkinson's Disease (IPD) is a progressive degenerative disorder of the nervous system, involving a reduction in the neurotransmitter dopamine from within the basal ganglia of the brain. The cause is unknown, but is likely to be a mix of genetic and environmental factors.

Most people are first diagnosed over the age of 50. It is more common in males than females, and there are estimated to be 120,000 people with IPD in the UK.

There are a number of conditions and medications that lead to similar symptoms; this is known as *Parkinsonism*.

3 Main characteristics of the condition

Symptoms in IPD are the same as in Parkinsonism, although the latter may not present with all of the symptoms. Medications may reduce some of the symptoms, while some appear only as the disease progresses. Symptoms may also vary on an hourly or daily basis. Symptoms include:

- muscle tremor at rest and in movement – particularly characteristic is a rubbing of the thumb and first two fingers in one hand;
- freezing of movement, making it difficult to move rapidly (bradykinesia);
- increased joint flexion in a rested position and kyphotic posture;
- poor gait, involving start hesitation and then hurrying with shortened, shuffling steps;
- postural instability, with associated risk and fear of falling;
- loss of facial expression, described as mask-like face (hypomimia);
- reduced volume and clarity of speech;
- dementia;
- depression.

4 Effects of the condition on exercise response

- Poor ability to control involuntary and voluntary movements (dyskinesia)
- Reduced ability to control speed, variety in speed and to immediately put commands into action
- Reduced range of movement
- Poor thermoregulation
- Accelerated heart rate and blood pressure responses
- Fear and risk of falling
- Reduced ability to interpret intensity from facial expression and talk testing

- Worsening of any of the above with increased intensity and/or duration

5 Medications and their effect on exercise response

All the medications are characterised by a gradual decrease in their effectiveness and a gradual increase in their side-effects, usually occurring approximately five years after the first prescription. Increasing amounts of the drug are prescribed to increase the effectiveness, but side-effects usually increase proportionally. Dopaminergics and anticholinergics, the two main groups of drugs, can all have rather severe side-effects. Effects on exercise response include:

- confusion;
- drowsiness;
- dizziness or fainting;
- further movement disorders.

6 Important rules

- Concentrate on eccentric rather than concentric contractions to avoid increasing kyphotic (rounded) posture and flexed positions in all joints
- Avoid the treadmill initially if there is a risk of falls
- Query whether additional medications are being taken to reduce side-effects; if so, investigate their side-effects
- Suggest the client liaises with their prescriber to find out if taking an altered dose at a specific time before exercise may improve exercise response
- Ensure water is available and maintain a comfortable temperature in the environment to aid in thermoregulation
- If hand tremor worsens, stop the exercise (keeping leg movement to avoid blood

Figure 3.22

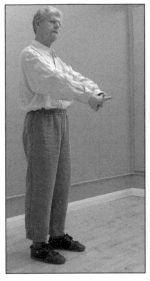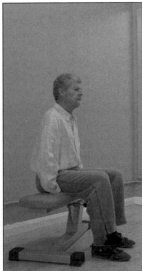

including their posture, gait, range of movement and reactions.

Include some active, dynamic stretches (see fig. 3.4 on pages 78–80) to encourage control of large movement. Use diagonal planes of movement where possible, to increase range and to work through life-related movements. Include mobility and pulse raising based on individual fitness.

CV

This should be based on individual fitness. Ensure it includes walking or running, as practise and feedback on gait may help to maintain or improve it.

Note any increased pulse rate response, taking longer to gradually raise pulse at the start, taking active rests during the maintenance and taking longer to gradually lower pulse at the end.

pooling if required) and hold a stretch for up to two minutes, as shown in figure 3.22
- If there is a slow response to instructions, be aware of the safety of others during off-the-spot exercises

7 Goals of the exercise programme

- Maintain or improve function for everyday life
- Maintain independence
- Maintain or improve gait to reduce fear and risk of falling
- Maintain or improve joint range
- Improve mood.

8 Programming principles

Warm-up

Use this as an opportunity to assess the individual's abilities at each exercise session,

Resistance

Include life-related movements, involving bodyweight and small equipment or cables rather than machines. Hard gripping may increase tremor, so encourage a looser grip or consider equipment that does not require high-grip tension, for example wrist weights or bands with loops.

Select strength or resistance bias according to individual goals. Work on range of movement and quality of movement before increasing repetitions or resistance.

Co-ordination

Introduce exercises that work on a variety of reaction and speed. Also include exercises that safely challenge co-ordination, including ball games and standing balance exercises. Provide feedback on standing/seated posture throughout. Increase the complexity of exercise by combining leg and arm movements after initially working them in isolation.

Cool-down and flexibility

Ensure a return to pre-exercise heart rate before commencing an extended flexibility component. Find the most comfortable positions for each stretch, before performing static development stretches followed by dynamic stretches in muscles crossing flexed joints. Non-affected joints should be stretched as for any individual.

9 Teaching principles

Allow additional time between reps and sets for processing of information into action. Ask for feedback and be prepared to use patience when waiting for responses. Note that talking and exercising may significantly increase the challenge of an exercise, but this can be useful as it reflects real life.

10 Personalise it!

Provide guidance related, for example, to the client's other medical conditions: goals; likes and dislikes; lifestyle.

1 Name of condition

Cerebral palsy (CP)

2 Definition and incidence of condition

Cerebral palsy is defined by non-progressive damage to the parts of the brain responsible for muscle tone and spinal reflexes. This damage occurs before, during or soon after birth. There are estimated to be 110,000 people with CP in the UK.

3 Main characteristics of the condition

CP affects people in many different ways and with differing severity. Characteristics include:

- muscle flaccidity, where there is a lack of tension in the muscles;
- muscle contractures/spasm, where there is too much tension in the muscles;
- difficulty in controlling voluntary movement, affecting balance and movement co-ordination;
- speech impairment, including difficulty with word articulation and voice volume;
- difficulty in controlling eye movement;
- difficulty in swallowing;
- other brain dysfunction, including learning disability.

4 Effects of the condition on exercise response

The CP-ISRA (Cerebral Palsy – International Sport and Recreation Association) uses a classification system from 1 to 8, based on functional ability, as follows:

- CP 1–4 designate a range of ability, from someone who has the inability to self-propel a wheelchair and no lower limb function or trunk stability, through to someone who can walk for short distances using aids but needs to sit to remain stable for most exercises;
- CP 5–8 refer to people who can exercise from a standing position, from someone who has spasticity significantly affecting function on one side of their upper and/or lower limbs, through to someone whose loss of function is minimal.

For those with greater impairment, the reduced mechanical efficiency and increased metabolic cost of controlled exercise is such that there may be up to a 50 per cent reduction in work capacity. Early fatigue is also therefore common. For those with minor impairment, the condition will have little impact on exercise response.

Spasticity may increase during an exercise session and for a short while after. This is not dangerous, but may cause distress. In the long term, exercise has been shown to decrease spasticity and therefore improve daily function.

5 Medications and their effect on exercise response

Anti-seizure and anti-spasmodic medications can affect concentration and motivation, and can cause depression. Anti-spasmodic medication is likely to reduce muscular strength. While this may enable greater control of smooth, efficient movements in affected muscles, it will at the same time reduce function in all muscles throughout the body.

6 Important rules

- Be ready to provide strapping and wrapping for assisting use of equipment, for example assisting with grip or keeping feet in pedals of bikes (see fig. 3.20 on page 115), being aware they may need to be quickly removed due to muscle spasm
- Never force joints that are locked as a result of muscle spasm

7 Goals of the exercise programme

- Improve function for daily living, including posture, balance and co-ordination
- Improve independence
- Prevent secondary diseases caused by lack of physical activity
- Provide social opportunities

8 Programming principles

Warm-up

Use this as an opportunity to assess daily function, including energy, concentration, motivation and spasticity, adjusting the remainder of the workout accordingly. Minimise challenge relating to balance and co-ordination to ensure these do not prevent effective pulse-raising. Ensure a very gradual increase is achieved, offering intermittent mobility exercises (for mobility and active rest) to enable a long warm-up (see page 71).

Avoid stretching muscles with low tone (loss of nerve input). Dynamic stretches may be effective for muscles with normal or high tone (too much nerve input), assisting body awareness.

CV

Consider using non-affected limbs on their own to enable a greater duration and intensity, while balancing this with exercise to improve function for walking/self-propelling a wheelchair. Encourage slow, controlled, flowing movements.

Resistance

Progress range of movement to aid in daily function before increasing resistance and repetitions. Strength-biased training may increase spasticity for the next few hours, but the functional benefits may outweigh any short-term effects for those who feel comfortable with this.

Resistance bands and cables are not only more functional, but provide greater feedback to the muscles for controlling eccentric contractions.

Co-ordination

Isolate challenging movements, particularly those required for ADLs. After working affected muscles in isolation, consider increasing the challenge by introducing compound exercises involving other muscles.

Walking involves complex, compound movement and becomes even more complex when on a treadmill. Set the challenge appropriately.

Cool-down and flexibility

Offer a re-warm before stretching if the client has cooled down during relatively small-range or muscle group exercises. Active stretches may be more effective than passive stretches (*see* pages 83–7).

9 Teaching principles

If the client has a tendency to dribble, do not assume they have a learning disability. The two are not necessarily related. Assess cognition separately from physical function and then communicate at an appropriate level.

Attempt to sit at eye level when communicating with the client if they are a wheelchair user.

10 Personalise it!

Provide guidance related, for example, to the client's other medical conditions; goals; likes and dislikes; lifestyle.

Metabolic conditions

Metabolic conditions are those in which the production of hormones and/or sensitivity to these hormones is compromised. They include type I and type II diabetes, and obesity.

See ACSM Position Stands on obesity and type II diabetes.

Immunological and haematological conditions

Immunological conditions are those in which the body is challenged in its ability to defend itself against viruses and bacteria. Haematological conditions can also affect the body's defence mechanisms, as well as affecting any organs or bodily functions dependent on a healthy blood supply.

1 Name of condition

Cancer

2 Definition and incidence of condition

Cancer is a term used to label over 200 different diseases, which all cause uncontrolled growth of abnormal cells and destruction of surrounding healthy tissue. The four most common cancers account for more than half of all cases. These cancers are breast, lung, bowel and prostate.

Primary cancer is the name given to the initial disease; *secondary* cancer is the name given to cancer that has spread (in the blood or lymph) to a new site.

There are estimated to be 1.2 million people alive in the UK who have had a diagnosis of cancer during their life.

3 Main characteristics of the condition

Each cancer has its own distinct set of characteristics. For example:

- Pain if there is a tumour in the musculoskeletal system;
- Breathlessness if there is a tumour in the lungs;
- Paralysis and seizures if there is a tumour in the brain;
- Fatigue.

4 Effects of the condition on exercise response

The effect on exercise response will be dependent on the area of the body affected. Commonly with many cancers, people experience low energy levels.

5 Medications and their effect on exercise response

Medications, especially chemotherapy and radiotherapy, can have severe side-effects. If the individual is experiencing illness from the side-effects of chemotherapy, they should obviously not be attending a fitness facility until after the end of the course of treatment. Radiotherapy can cause skin irritation made worse by perspiration. Other common side-effects include pain, muscle weakness, and fatigue.

Short-term and long-term side effects of chemotherapy, radiotherapy and other medications should be noted separately.

6 Important rules

- Liaise with the client's consultant to ensure the proposed exercise programme is not likely to increase the risk of secondaries (new sites for the cancer cells)
- There should be no massage (unless by an appropriately qualified and advised practitioner), or taking of blood pressure on the side of the body affected by the cancer

7 Goals of the exercise programme

- Reduced fatigue
- Maintenance in bodyweight
- Maintenance or improvement in range of movement across affected joints
- Improved mood

8 Programming principles

Principles should depend on whether the cancer is localised or has spread to other sites, as well as the stage of the disease: first diagnosis; mid-treatment; remission. After diagnosis, and especially mid-treatment, there may need to be a reduced frequency, intensity and duration.

The priority of CV or resistance training is dependent on the type of cancer.

Consider adaptation within each component according to the site of the cancer and its impact on exercise response.

9 Personalise it!

Provide guidance related, for example, to the client's other medical conditions, goals, likes and dislikes, and lifestyle.

---

1 Name of condition

Fibromyalgia

2 Definition and incidence of condition

Of unknown cause, *fibromyalgia* affects many body systems, presenting as chronic pain and tenderness, diagnosed by a medical practitioner testing the presence of these at a range of specific anatomic sites. It affects muscles and ligaments but not the joint capsule.

It affects 2.5 million people in the UK, with approximately 80 per cent of these being women. Diagnoses are increasing as medical practitioners become increasingly familiar with the diagnostic tools available. From 1990 to 2001, diagnoses increased by 35 per cent.

3 Main characteristics of the condition

Fibromyalgia is characterised by pain, chronic fatigue, numbness at the extremities, disturbed sleep, morning muscle stiffness, depression and anxiety.

4 Effects of the condition on exercise response

Anxiety and fear that exercise will worsen the condition often create a barrier to participation in active living, let alone more formal exercise. There may also be difficulty in controlling eccentric muscle contractions, a greater muscle soreness response and a longer recovery time than would usually be expected.

5 Medications and their effect on exercise response

Medications are unlikely to have any adverse impact on exercise response. Pain suppressants and antidepressants may increase the success of a new exercise programme.

6 Important rules

- Progressing the programme too quickly could cause a worsening of the condition. Liaise carefully with the client to ensure an appropriate rate of progression
- Use an RPE scale to monitor pain and another to monitor fatigue (*see* page xx), noting daily variations. Keep a record of daily variations to see if a pattern emerges
- Avoid early-morning exercise; late morning is often the best time to exercise
- Since early drop-out rates tend to be high (due to short-term increases in pain, fear of the conditioning worsening and depression), extra time may need to be spent with the client in order to support and motivate them. Encourage social interaction, especially with other clients who have conditions causing pain and/or who have an empathetic nature

7 Goals of the exercise programme

- Decreased pain
- Improved sleep
- Increased energy levels
- Improved mood
- Prevention of secondary diseases caused by lack of physical activity

8 Programming principles

Warm-up

Use this as an opportunity to assess daily function, including pain, energy and motivation, adjusting the remainder of the workout accordingly. On bad days, the workout could consist of flexibility and relaxation only, while on good days it could consist of all components.

Ensure a long warm-up is achieved, using whatever pulse-raising activity causes the least pain.

CV

Increase duration before intensity. Avoid high impact activities.

Resistance

Emphasise concentric contractions (usually lifting a weight), minimising eccentric contractions (usually lowering a weight). Use endurance-biased training, rather than strength training. Minimise repetitions of activities above shoulder height, which can increase pain.

Co-ordination

Include functional activities for everyday life, such as squats, turning and so on.

Cool-down and flexibility

Use this as an opportunity to encourage relaxation. Consider finding a quiet area to enable the success of a relaxation session. Static, passive stretches will aid relaxation and may decrease pain.

9 Teaching principles

Patience and empathy may be required in abundance! Use techniques that may limit drop-out, including phoning anyone who misses two or more successive sessions.

10 Personalise it!

Provide guidance related, for example, to the client's other medical conditions, goals, likes and dislikes, and lifestyle.

1 Name of condition

HIV and AIDS (Human immuno-deficiency virus and Acquired immune deficiency syndrome)

2 Definition and incidence of condition

AIDS is a progressive disease caused by the suppression of elements (CD4 cells) within the body's immune system.

In 2000 there were estimated to be 36 million adults worldwide infected with HIV. In the UK, in 2003, there were 57,000 cases of HIV diagnosed, plus likely to be 14,500 people undiagnosed. Two-thirds of heterosexual diagnoses were in women (UK Health Protection Agency).

3 Main characteristics of the condition

There are three stages of HIV – in Stage I, there are no symptoms, but in Stage II symptoms become apparent and include:

- increased risk and incidence of infection;
- decreased lean body mass and body tissue wastage, causing weight loss;
- decreased appetite;
- fatigue;
- peripheral neuropathy (damage to nerve endings);
- depression and anxiety.

In Stage III, when there is severe depletion of disease-fighting cells, the above symptoms become more severe. Additionally, secondary diseases, often caused by viral infection, are common, including cancer.

Not all people infected by HIV progress from Stage I and it is common for people to remain asymptomatic for 10 years or more.

4 Effects of the condition on exercise response

For those who are in Stage I, there is no change in exercise response. As symptoms start and progress, the metabolic cost of exercise increases. Common reasons for this include reduced CV capacity (due to respiratory and lung infections), pain, fatigue and depression. Energy levels may vary considerably.

5 Medications and their effect on exercise response

Medications vary greatly in their effect, from having no effect to causing weight loss, anaemia (reducing the oxygen-carrying capacity of the blood) and a rapid heart rate.

Some medications may have an effect on fat distribution, increasing fat deposits around the trunk and neck and decreasing it around the arms and face. Exercise is unlikely to alter this.

6 Important rules

- A sudden change in health status and/or in exercise tolerance is a contra-indication to exercise
- A new exercise regime should be commenced during a period of relatively good health
- Low- to moderate-intensity exercise is known to boost immunity, while high-intensity exercise is known to suppress immunity. Therefore, avoid high-intensity exercise
- Follow additional advice for secondary conditions, for example cancer

7 Goals of the exercise programme

- Increase immunity (low- to moderate-intensity exercise only).
- Maintain and/or improve lean muscle mass
- Maintain and/or improve energy levels
- Maintain and/or improve mood
- Maintain and/or improve appetite

8 Programming principles

If energy levels are low, people may prefer to participate in low-intensity exercise that promotes relaxation, such as tai chi, yoga or stretch. These have been shown to improve mood and boost immunity. If time has been taken off due to ill-health, it is important to restart at a lower intensity and rebuild it very gradually.

If the individual wishes to participate in general exercise classes or the gym:

Warm-up

A very gradual increase in intensity is advised to ensure immunity is not negatively impacted upon.

CV

Use low- to moderate-intensity maintenance or interval training, for no longer than 30 minutes. Durations above this have been shown to risk increasing undesired weight loss.

Resistance

This is often the most important component of the exercise programme. Muscular strength-biased training is recommended, to aid weight maintenance/gain.

Cool-down and flexibility

A very gradual decrease in intensity is advised to ensure immunity is not negatively impacted upon. Offer a suitable area for relaxation.

10 Personalise it!

Provide guidance related, for example, to the client's other medical conditions, goals, likes and dislikes, and lifestyle.

Cognitive and psychological conditions

Cognitive and psychological conditions are those resulting from alterations in brain chemistry, make-up and function.

1 Name of condition

Down's Syndrome (DS)

2 Definition and incidence of condition

Down's Syndrome is a genetic condition caused by an extra chromosome (chromosome 21), which causes specific physical characteristics and a learning disability.

There are estimated to be 60,000 people with DS in the UK population.

3 Main characteristics of the condition

- Characteristic facial features include flattened features, slanted eyes, smaller nose and smaller mouth
- Shorter height
- Tendency to hearing and/or visual impairment
- Low IQ (often moderate learning disability, with IQ of 35-50; normative being set at 70 and average for the population being 100)
- Difficulty understanding and interpreting information
- Communication difficulties, including speaking, reading and writing
- Tendency to epilepsy
- Heart defects (affects 40 per cent of people with DS)

- Tendency to hypertension
- Tendency to hypothyroidism – causing lethargy and weight gain
- Increased joint laxity/hypermobility, including atlanto-axial instability (hypermobility at the top of the vertebral column; affects 17 per cent of people with DS)
- Tendency to osteoarthritis
- Physical conditioning difficulties
- Tendency to obesity
- Tendency to be overly friendly and affectionate.

4 Effects of the condition on exercise response

- Reduced comprehension
- Reduced ability to communicate (including reading letters and numbers)
- Reduced cardiovascular capacity, including that due to a lower maximal heart rate
- Ability to perform too large a range of movement

5 Medications and their effect on exercise response

Anti-hypertensive medications may prevent the heart rate increasing relative to exercise intensity. Use RPE instead of pulse-rate monitoring. Anti-convulsants may cause drowsiness and reduced concentration.

6 Important rules

- Patience!
- Ensure a legal advocate countersigns the PAR-Q if the client does not have legal consent.
- Ask whether the client has atlanto-axial instability, whereby there is hypermobility at the top of the neck. If the client does have it, extreme caution should be taken to avoid use

of the available range (which could possibly cause death), including avoidance of high-impact activities

- Individuals often find routine helpful. This should be respected and encompassed within any new exercise programme
- Attempt to include tools to encourage independence including adapted RPE scales (see table 3.2 on page 69)
- Never stretch hyperflexible muscles
- Be prepared to use alternative forms of communication, including Makaton or Sign Supported English (see pages 101–3)
- Set clear boundaries for acceptable behaviour, both in terms of the client with you and the client with other facility users. This should be dealt with firmly but thoughtfully

7 Goals of the exercise programme

- Increase confidence
- Improve social skills
- Improve body awareness
- Prevent secondary diseases caused by lack of physical activity

8 Programming principles

It may be necessary to keep to the same programme to assist with recognition and ownership. Progression may be slower than physical capability allows, as it may be influenced by comprehension and memory as much as by physical progress.

Warm-up

Include the idea that concentration should be warmed up, just as much as the physical body. Do not stretch hyperflexible muscles. Use mobility exercises to set safe ranges of movement in hypermobile joints.

CV

Offer a range of different modes if attention span is low. Move swiftly from one exercise to the next to build duration. Consider using the numbers and pictures on CV machine consoles, or music in the studio, to aid concentration.

Due to cardiovascular limitations, heart rate monitoring and use of conventional formulae for heart rate ranges may be inappropriate. Increase duration before intensity.

The treadmill might be an inappropriate mode until there is sufficient confidence, body awareness and concentration.

Resistance Training

Use resistance machines or lightweight equipment (such as bands) to reduce risk while the client is initially learning about safe use of equipment. Work towards strength-biased training in hypermobile joints, to reduce hypermobility.

Encourage control of eccentric contractions if there is a tendency to rush.

To aid concentration, consider using a circuit approach when there are two or more sets to be performed – that is, complete one set of each exercise before repeating the sequence again.

Co-ordination

Consider including fun games that improve motor skills.

Cool-down and flexibility

Include an activity that promotes calm if the exercise has increased excitement. Avoid any stretching of hyperflexible muscles.

9 Teaching principles

Be prepared to repeat your instructions as if you were teaching the programme for the first time, rather than the tenth time.

Use pictures and symbols on a programme card to assist with recognition and memory, for example pictures of exercises cut from a magazine, or ◆ (diamond), ⊙ (spot), ■ (square) ✻ (star) instead of conventional names for exercises.

Consider your standing position, using it to cut off the surrounding environment if the client finds it difficult to maintain focus. Standing in front of the client and shadowing the movement required while they perform it allows copying of pace and range of movement to aid safety and understanding. Use non-conventional RPE scales to monitor exercise intensity.

Avoid using 'right' and 'left' for directional instructions, using items in the environment instead, for example the door, the window, the stereo, etc.

Gain client feedback by asking closed and open questions. If the client has a tendency to say 'yes' in answer to questioning (because they want to please), rephrase your questions to assist in gaining more accurate answers.

Consider the best use of the carers/friends who attend to support and motivate the client, if possible training them safely and effectively to instruct specific exercises. Attempt to reduce the level of supervision as appropriate to the individual, from direct one-to-one working, to observing from a distance, to being available for occasional support.

10 Personalise it!

Provide guidance related, for example, to the client's other medical conditions, goals, likes and dislikes, and lifestyle.

1 Name of condition

Mental illness

2 Definition and incidence of condition

Mental illness is a term used to cover a range of different behavioural, biological or psychological conditions that affect ability to function, including depression, bi-polar disorder, schizophrenia and disorders due to substance abuse.

Up to 30 per cent of all visits to a GP are linked to a mental health problem. Up to 1.5 per cent of the population have a chronic (long-term) mental health problem. Disabled people are at a higher risk of mental illness secondary to another condition.

3 Main characteristics of the condition

Mental illness involves dysfunction in the areas of emotion, mood and/or personality. Characteristics include:

- mania (unusually high energy and mood);
- depression (unusually low energy and mood, feelings of sadness);
- psychosis (loss of contact with reality);
- anxiety (overwhelming sense of apprehension or fear);
- inability to adhere to social norms.

Mental illness may arise as a condition secondary to a primary condition.

4 Effects of the condition on exercise response

- Low motivation or over-enthusiasm, or interchangeable between these
- Poor attendance or ability to attend at set appointment times
- Low concentration
- Poor body awareness
- Poor ability to process information

- Type of environment may increase risk of panic attacks

5 Medications and their effect on exercise response

While some medications will enable the individual to function at a social level, others will dull the senses, both emotional and physical. As with all medications, response time from the initial dose varies, in this case, from a few hours to three weeks.

Medications may cause sedation, blunting all responses. Other effects on exercise response include:

- low concentration;
- confusion;
- agitation;
- poor balance;
- weight gain;
- dry mouth;
- tremor;
- increased sweating;
- increased/unstable blood pressure;
- changes in heart rhythm.

6 Important rules

- Ensure that clients are compliant with their medication. Those who believe they are feeling so well that their medication is no longer required may stop taking it, leading to sudden onset of ill-health that may put themselves and/or others at risk
- Attempt to involve the client in as much of the decision-making as possible
- Ask the client about the effect of exercise mode, time of day and changes in mood

7 Goals of the exercise programme

- Improvement in mood
- Social opportunity
- Improvement in self-esteem
- Provision of a sense of purpose
- Improved management of anger, distress and psychological function
- Distraction from negative factors
- Prevention of secondary diseases caused by lack of physical activity

8 Programming principles

As for a non-disabled person, the programme should be appropriate to fitness level and personalised goals. Additionally, warm-up and cool-down may need to be extended to aid mood and concentration. Relaxation may be a relatively important component and therefore exercise with a spiritual element, such as yoga, may be appropriate.

9 Teaching principles

Show patience in communication. Consider strategies to deal with lack of motivation, poor attendance or early drop-out.

10 Personalise it!

Provide guidance related, for example, to the client's other medical conditions, goals, likes and dislikes, and lifestyle.

1 Name of condition

Dementia

2 Definition and incidence of condition

Dementia is a term used to describe a range of brain conditions affecting memory, mood, thinking and communication. There are two categories of dementia:

- progressive/degenerative, for example Alzheimer's Disease;
- non-progressive, for example as a result of a stroke.

There are believed to be 750,000 people living with dementia, only 18,000 of these being under the age of 65.

3 Main characteristics of the condition

These will vary according to the type of dementia, but typically include:

- loss of memory, often short-term memory;
- agitation;
- confusion;
- depression;
- difficulty with forming a sentence;
- sudden changes in mood and emotional expression, including anger and physical aggression.

In the latter stages, physical impairments are common, such as an inability to control voluntary movements.

4 Effects of the condition on exercise response

- Low motivation
- Poor attendance or ability to attend at set appointment times
- Low concentration
- Poor body awareness
- Poor balance
- Poor ability to process information

- Reduced control of conscious movement
- Early fatigue

5 Medications and their effect on exercise response

Commonly prescribed drugs can cause:

- low concentration;
- poor balance;
- dry mouth;
- tremor;
- increased sweating;
- increased/unstable blood pressure;
- changes in heart rhythm.

6 Important rules

- Offer a consistent programme to allow information to be absorbed into long-term memory
- Ensure exercise complexity is appropriate and not so challenging as to cause distress or confusion
- Patience
- Morning can often be a preferable time to exercise
- If the client is a risk to themselves or others, home exercise may be more appropriate than a facility-based programme

7 Goals of the exercise programme

- Maintenance of independence
- Improvement in self-esteem
- Provision of social opportunity
- Distraction from negative factors

8 Programming principles

These will be very dependent on the individual's level of comprehension. In the early stages a programme that you may use for a non-disabled person is likely to be appropriate. As the dementia progresses, the programme will need to become shorter and simpler, with the main focus being on ADLs (for example, walking) and fun.

CV

Duration may be limited by the level of concentration that can be maintained. Aim to maintain continuous activity for as long as concentration will allow, even if this means use of several different modes. Use an RPE scale most suited to the individual (see table 3.2 on page 69).

Resistance

If there is a risk that free weights will be dropped, use resistance machines or resistance bands. Isolation exercises, involving only one joint, may become increasingly more suitable, as they involve lower levels of co-ordination.

9 Teaching principles

Be patient in communication, and be prepared to teach the same programme with little progression for a long period, in order for the client to maintain familiarity with their exercise programme and be at ease within the facility.

Consider strategies to deal with lack of motivation, poor attendance or early drop-out. Encourage attendance by a carer who has an interest in motivating and supporting the client.

Be prepared for sudden changes in emotion, realising that any expression of anger should not be taken personally by the instructor.

10 Personalise it!

Provide guidance related, for example, to the client's other medical conditions, goals, likes and dislikes, and lifestyle.

Sensory conditions

Sensory conditions are those affecting hearing, sight, touch or smell.

1 Name of condition

Hearing impairment

2 Definition and incidence of condition

Hearing impairment covers a range of conditions that result in a reduced ability to hear, from partial loss through to complete deafness. Fifty per cent of deafness is of unknown cause.

There are nine million deaf or hard of hearing people in the UK.

3 Main characteristics of the condition

The condition involves loss of hearing ability. People with hearing impairment may use an assistive hearing device (hearing-aid), lip-reading and/or sign language.

4 Effects of the condition on exercise response

Hearing impairment is unlikely to affect exercise response, other than when balance is challenged. However, low confidence may affect willingness to start and maintain an exercise programme.

5 Medications and their effect on exercise response

Medication is rarely prescribed for long-term hearing loss.

6 Important rules

Find out how the client would prefer to communicate (*see* page xx), for example:

- using their hearing-aid and the facility's hearing induction loop;
- lip-reading;
- Sign Supported English;
- British Sign Language (via an interpreter).

Whenever you speak to the person, ensure you face them in order to assist with lip-reading. Use a hearing induction loop if the client has an appropriate setting on their hearing-aid.

While some deaf people will enjoy feeling the vibrations created by loud music, others will feel nauseous. It is therefore important to consult about music.

Facilities should have an emergency alarm system with flashing lights. In an emergency, remember to evacuate those who are not in a position to see that evacuation is required.

Some deaf people prefer to be in the company of other deaf people. Consider offering an exercise session (gym or studio-based) specifically for this group.

7 Goals of the exercise programme

- Improve self-esteem
- Increase social interaction
- Prevention of secondary diseases caused by lack of physical activity

8 Programming principles

Programming principles should be applied as for any non-disabled person, or taking into account any other medical conditions. In some cases, balance and spatial awareness will be affected, so should be appropriately challenged within the programme.

9 Teaching principles

Adapt the teaching technique used to introduce new exercises as required by the client. Position yourself carefully so that your face and any demonstrations can be seen.

10 Personalise it!

Provide guidance related, for example, to the client's other medical conditions, goals, likes and dislikes, and lifestyle.

---

1 Name of condition

Visual impairment

2 Definition and incidence of condition

Visual impairment covers many conditions, both primary and secondary, which have caused partial sight through to complete blindness. Only approximately five per cent of visually impaired people have no light perception at all.

There are estimated to be two million visually impaired people in the UK, the vast majority of these being over the age of 65.

3 Main characteristics of the condition

Visual impairment ranges from reduced through to complete loss of light perception, causing:

- Loss of sharpness – fuzzy objects;
- Loss of field – loss of width/height of what can be seen – vision through a specific area only;
- Loss of depth – loss of distance perception;
- Loss of colour – tone brightness or colour perception.

4 Effects of the condition on exercise response

Although visual impairment in itself does not affect exercise response, there may be a primary condition causing the visual impairment that does affect it.

Those with a significant visual impairment, especially those who have had it since childhood, may have poor posture, poor body awareness, reduced balance and a low fitness level caused by lack of physical activity.

5 Medications and their effect on exercise response

Note medications given for the primary condition.

6 Important rules

- Ensure glasses/contact lenses owned by the client are worn within the exercise environment to make the most of any sight
- Offer a guided tour of the facilities, pointing out raised signage and how to find these signs
- Offer large-print, Braille or recorded options for all printed material and for recording the individual's exercise programme
- When guiding a blind person, offer your arm for them to hold. They may walk one pace behind you. Inform them of any changes in surface, including stairs, before walking on them
- Ensure there are no trip hazards and that any changes in the usual environment are reported to regular users
- If the person comes with a guide dog, ensure the assistance dog policy is followed. It is not appropriate to allow the dog to stand alongside the individual while they exercise. A suitable area should be found in a quiet area of the gym or outside the exercise studio
- Once the person becomes familiar with the environment, they should be able to exercise independently, possibly except when setting up certain machinery

7 Goals of the exercise programme

- Prevention of secondary diseases caused by lack of physical activity
- Improved posture

8 Programming principles

Programming principles should be applied as for any non-disabled person, or taking into account the primary condition. Additionally:

Co-ordination

Without visual feedback, balance may be poor. Although use of the treadmill is not necessarily impossible, it does provide a high level of challenge especially if running. Working on standing balance, posture and body awareness will assist with daily life.

9 Teaching principles

Adapt the teaching technique used to introduce new exercises, as demonstrations may be pointless. Provide sufficient initial instructions and teaching points for safety, then talk the client into position and provide feedback to maximise effectiveness.

Consider the order of exercises in the gym environment for independence in moving between exercises, as well as effective overload.

10 Personalise it!

Provide guidance related, for example, to the client's other medical conditions, goals, likes and dislikes, and lifestyle.

SUMMARY

20

By taking extra time in the planning and preparation stages, you and your clients have an increased opportunity to work together successfully. Consultation with your clients at every stage increases the opportunity for them to take ownership of their own exercise programme and absorb it into their lifestyle.

Keep reminding yourself that you should always be able to answer questions that start with *why*, *what* and *how*:

- Why does this client want to exercise?
- What do I do and what does this client need to know to ensure safety?
- What exercises is this client going to do and why?
- How am I going to instruct?
- How am I going to ensure effective progression?

The more involvement your client has in answering these questions and the greater their understanding, the more empowered they are likely to feel.

Be prepared to adapt your programming and instructing to take on board your client's feedback and to create an appropriate level of challenge at each and every workout.

APPENDIX I STEP-BY-STEP ACTION PLAN FOR SAFE, EFFECTIVE TRAINING WITH DISABLED PEOPLE

Use 'sense-able', client-centred communication for feedback at every step

Show around
Draw attention to those images/sounds/sensations with which they most identify.

PAR-Q
Offer assistance where required and probe 'yes' answers. Refer positive PAR-Q to medically qualified practitioner, liaising as required. Await written consent, carefully reading it to ensure consent is granted and take on board any recommendations.

Qualified?
Are you qualified to work with this individual? Is there someone better qualified than you within your facility? Do you know who to refer to if there is no qualified person within your facility?

Questions
Ask questions about function, lifestyle, goals, likes/dislikes. Involve participants (and carers/interpreters).

Functional assessment
Take assessment measures related to current function and goals, to enable programming, monitoring of progress and motivation.

Research

Use the tools that are available (the client, colleagues, medically trained acquaintances, and the internet) to research medical conditions and medications.

Write programme

Using all the information gained, prepare a programme, ensuring it includes information on all FITTA principles. Consider whether more than one programme is required.

Induction

Introduce the client to the programme, altering type where required, setting precise intensities and times, and offering the opportunity for feedback throughout.

Monitoring

Consider how to encourage independence and ownership of the programme. Consider best use of carers and other facility users.

Evaluation

Alter the programme whenever client feedback suggests changes are required. At least every six weeks offer a functional reassessment and revisit goals.

APPENDIX 2 SAMPLE PRO-FORMA FOR BASIS OF INDIVIDUAL APPROACH TO TRAINING

NAME OF CLIENT:

Definition

Main characteristics

Effects of the condition on exercise response

Medications

Rules

Goals

Programming principles

Teaching principles

Personal information

GLOSSARY

Acute	Short term
ADLs	Activities of daily living
Bilateral	Both sides of the body
CV	Cardiovascular
Chronic	Long term
Contralateral	Opposite sides of the body
Disability	Loss or limitation of opportunity to participate in everyday life, as a result of one or more barriers
Empowerment	Personalised control over decision-making by an individual
Exercise	Formal, planned physical activity that is over and above the requirements of daily living
Extrinsic	Relating to factors outside the individual
Fitness	The ability to perform vigorous physical activity
Gait	Walking technique
Hyper	Too much
Hypo	Too little
IFI	Inclusive Fitness Initiative
Impairment	Medical condition
Intrinsic	Relating to factors inside the individual
Ipsilateral	Same sides of the body
Kyphotic	Exaggerated curvature of the thoracic spine, causing a rounded posture
Mechanical efficiency	The energy efficiency of a selected movement pathway
Metabolic cost	Energy expenditure, measured in units, e.g. calories
Paralysis	Loss of nerve connection between the brain and the body
Paresis	Partial paralysis
Physical activity	Any movement created by skeletal muscles that requires energy expenditure
REPs	Register of Exercise Professionals
RPE	Rate of perceived exertion
Unilateral	One side of the body

REFERENCES AND FURTHER READING

American College of Sports Medicine (1998), The recommended quantity and quality of exercise for developing and maintaining cardiorespiratory and muscular fitness, and flexibility in healthy adults, *Medicine and Science in Sports and Exercise*, 30(6):976–991.

American College of Sports Medicine (1998), Exercise and physical activity for older adults, *Medicine and Science in Sports and Exercise*, 30(6):992–1008.

American College of Sports Medicine (2001), Appropriate intervention strategies for weight loss and prevention of weight regain for adults, *Medicine and Science in Sports and Exercise*, 33(12):2145–2156.

American College of Sports Medicine (2004), Exercise and hypertension, *Medicine and Science in Sports and Exercise*, 36(3):533–553.

American College of Sports Medicine (2005), *Guidelines for Exercise Testing and Prescription*, Lippincott, Williams and Wilkins.

Borg, G.A. (1973), Perceived exertion: a note on history and methods, *Medicine and Science in Sports and Exercise*, 5(2):90–93.

Bouchard, C., Shephard, R.J. and Stephens, T. (1993), *Physical Activity, Fitness and Health*, Human Kinetics.

British Association of Cardiac Rehabilitation (2000), *Phase IV Exercise Instructor Training Module, revised edition*.

British Medical Association (2005), *Concise Guide to Medicines and Drugs*, Dorling Kindersley.

British National Formulary (Biannual), *Reference on Classified Notes on Clinical Conditions, Drugs and Preparations for Practitioners*, British Medical Association and Royal Pharmaceutical Society of Great Britain.

Chief Medical Office (2004), *At Least Five a Week: Evidence on the Impact of Physical Activity and its Relationship to Health*, HMSO.

Department of Health (2001), *Exercise Referral Systems: A National Quality Assurance Framework*, HMSO.

Department of Health (2004), *Choosing Health: Making Healthy Choices Easier*, HMSO.

Department of Health (2001), *Exercise Referral Systems: A National Quality Assurance Framework*, HMSO.

Department of Health (2000), *Health Survey for England 1998*, HMSO.

Department of Health (2001), *Valuing People: A New Strategy for Learning Disabilities for the 21st Century*, HMSO.

Durstine, J.L. and Moore, G.E. (2003), *ACSM's Exercise Management for Persons with Chronic Diseases and Disabilities*, Human Kinetics.

Haskell, W.L. (1994), Health consequences of physical activity: understanding challenges regarding dose-response, *Medicine and Science in Sports and Exercise*, 26(6):649–660.

Health and Safety Executive (2003), *Five Steps to Risk Assessment*, HMSO.

Institute of Medicine of the National Academies (2005), *Workshop on Disability in America, a New Look*, National Academies Press.

Kasser, S.L. and Lytle, R.K. (2005), *Inclusive Physical Activity: A Lifetime of Opportunities*, Human Kinetics.

Later Life Training (2006), *Specialist Postural Stability Instructor Training Manual, revised edition*.

Mehrabian, A. (1981), *Silent Messages: Implicit Communication of Emotions and Attitudes*, Wadsworth.

Mental Health Foundation (2005), *Up and Running*, Mental Health Foundation.

Miller, W. and Rollink, S. (2002), *Motivational Interviewing: Preparing People for Change*, The Guilford Press.

Norris, C. (2000), *Back Stability*, Human Kinetics.

O'Connor, J. and McDermott, I. (2001), *Way of NLP*, Thorsons.

Scottish Executive (2005), *Delivering for Health: Building a Health Service Fit for the Future*, HMSO.

Shephard, R.J. (1990), *Fitness in Special Populations*, Human Kinetics.

Schoeni, R.F., Martin, L.G., Andreski, P.M. and Freedman, V.A. (2005), Persistent and growing socioeconomic disparities in disability among the elderly: 1982–2002, *American Journal of Public Health*, 95(11): 2065–2070.

Sigal, R.J., Kenny, G.P., Wasserman, D.H., Astandea-Sceppa, C. and White, R.D. (2006), Physical activity/exercise and type 2 diabetes: a consensus statement from the American Diabetes Association, *Diabetes Care*, 29 (6):1433–1438.

Skelton, D., Dinan, S., Campbell, M. and Rutherford, O. (2005), Tailored group exercise (falls management exercise – FaME) reduces falls in community-dwelling older frequent fallers, *Age and Ageing*, 34(6): 636–639.

Sport England (2005), *Understanding Participation in Sport: A Systematic Review*, Sport England.

US Department of Health and Human Sciences (2000), *Healthy People 2010: Understanding and Improving Health*, 2nd edition, Washington DC: US Government Printing Office.

Van Hoof, S. (2005), *Leading Exercise and Activity in a Mental Health Setting*, YMCA Fitness Industry Training.

Ward, P., Wicebloom, S., Holmes, S. and Dinan, S. (2005), *Inclusive Health, Fitness and Activity: Disability*, YMCA Fitness Industry Training.

Willis, J.D. and Campbell, L.F. (1992), *Exercise Psychology*, Human Kinetics.

Wilmore J.H. and Costill, D.L. (2004), *Physiology of Sport and Exercise, 3rd edition*, Human Kinetics.

USEFUL WEBSITES

Aidsmap
www.aidsmap.com

Alzheimer's Society
www.alzheimers.org.uk

Arthritis Care
www.arthritiscare.org.uk

Association for Spina Bifida and Hydrocephalus
www.asbah.demon.co.uk

Autistic Society
www.nas.org.uk

Brain and Spine Foundation
www.brainandspine.org.uk

British Dyslexia Association
www.bda-dyslexia.org.uk

British National Formulary
www.bnf.org

British Medical Journal
www.bmj.com

Canadian Society for Exercise Physiology – for PAR-Q
www.csep.ca/

Department of Health
www.dh.gov.uk

Disability Now
www.disabilitynow.org.uk

Disability Rights Commission
www.drc-gb.org

Downs Syndrome Association
www.downs-syndrome.org.uk

English Federation of Disability Sport
www.efds.co.uk

Equal Adventure
www.equaladventure.co.uk

Inclusive Fitness Initiative
www.inclusivefitness.org.uk

Information on public services for disabled people
www.direct.gov.uk/disability

Information on medical conditions
www.prodigy.nhs.uk

Limbless Association
www.limbless-association.org

Mencap
www.mencap.org.uk

MIND
www.mind.org.uk

Multiple Sclerosis Society
www.mss.org.uk

MS Society
www.mssociety.org.uk

National Centre for Physical Activity for People with Disability
www.ncpad.org

National Osteoporosis Society
www.nos.org.uk

NICE
www.nice.org.uk

Parkinson's Disease Society
www.parkinsons.org.uk

RADAR
www.radar.org.uk

RNIB
www.rnib.org.uk

RNID
www.rnid.org.uk

Scope (for people with cerebral palsy)
www.scope.org.uk

Sense
www.sense.org.uk

Spinal Injuries Association
www.spinal.org.uk

Sport England
www.sportengland.org

Stroke Association
www.stroke.org.uk

Transport for London
www.tfl.gov.uk

YMCA Fitness Industry Training
www.ymcafit.org.uk

INDEX

Page numbers in italics show illustrations.

V
visual impairment 3, 143–4

W
warm-up 70, 71–7
  and arthritis 115
  and cerebral palsy 131
  and Down's Syndrome 138
  and fibromyalgia 134
  and HIV/AIDS 136
  and limb amputation 119
  and MS 127
  and osteoporosis 117
  and Parkinson's Disease 129
  and spinal cord injury 121
  stretching exercises 72–7, *73–5*, *78–80*
  and stroke/CVA 124

NOTES

NOTES

NOTES

NOTES

ALSO AVAILABLE IN THE *FITNESS PROFESSIONALS* SERIES

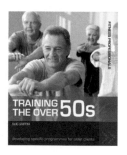

Training the Over 50s

The 50-plus age range has one of the fastest growing groups of regular gym-goers, who are increasingly turning to fitness instructors for guidance. Sue Griffin – a health promotions consultant who specialises in writing education programmes for adults and specialist populations – explains the relationship between fitness and ageing, and gives advice on training adults with chronic conditions and designing individual programmes. Packed with photographs and illustrations, this is the definitive handbook for any fitness professional working with older adults.

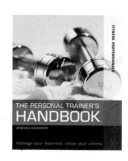

The Personal Trainer's Handbook

Whether you are newly qualified and looking for guidance on setting up your business or an established trainer looking for ideas to develop your company, this book will provide you with all the information you need. Rebecca Weissbort – a practising fitness trainer who has been involved in developing national standards for the fitness industry's governing body – gives invaluable advice on essential business skills, meeting clients' specific needs, and many other aspects of the personal training industry.

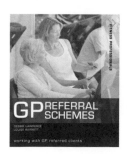

GP Referral Schemes

More and more, general practitioners are recognising the benefits of physical exercise in the treatment of many conditions. In this highly practical book, Debbie Lawrence (a highly regarded fitness expert) and Louise Barnett (a cardiac exercise specialist at London's King's College Hospital) provide everything you need to manage a referred client, including guidance on work planning for different types of client and differing levels of physical and behavioural change. An invaluable resource for any fitness professional working – or wishing to work – in the referrals sector of the industry.

Available from all good bookshops or online. For more details on these and other A&C Black sport and fitness titles, please go to www.acblack.com.